Killer Fat

Killer Fat

Media, Medicine, and Morals in the American "Obesity Epidemic"

NATALIE BOERO

RUTGERS UNIVERSITY PRESS

NEW BRUNSWICK, NEW JERSEY, AND LONDON

LIBRARY OF CONGRESS CATALOGING-IN-PUBLICATION DATA

Boero, Natalie, 1974–
    Killer fat : media, medicine, and morals in the American "obesity epidemic" /
Natalie Boero.
        p. cm.
    Includes bibliographical references and index.
    ISBN 978–0–8135–5371–9 (hardcover : alk. paper) — ISBN 978–0–8135–5372–6
(e-book)
    1. Obesity—Social aspects—United States.   2. Obesity—United States—
Psychological aspects.   3. Health in mass media.   4. Body image.   I. Title.
    RC552.O25B64   2012
    369.196'398—dc23
                                                                    2011046939

A British Cataloging-in-Publication record for this book is available
from the British Library.

Visit our website: http://rutgerspress.rutgers.edu

Manufactured in the United States of America

For Kristin and Raka

CONTENTS

ACKNOWLEDGMENTS

It is difficult to think of all the people I have to thank for helping this book come to fruition, but it is easy to think of whom to thank first. Without the generosity of my interviewees and all the various people I observed and spoke with, this book would simply not exist. To them I owe an immense debt of gratitude for sharing their stories and struggles with me and for allowing me to enter their lives. It is my sincere hope that I have represented their words and stories fairly.

It is almost an exercise in futility to find words to express my gratitude and sheer adoration of the two people to whom this book is dedicated, Kristin Barker and Raka Ray. Both have been exceptional mentors and friends and have believed in me and this project since its inception. Both have challenged me as a sociologist, taught me to take criticism, and have had an unparalleled impact on my intellectual and personal development for nearly twenty years. While Raka helped shape earlier versions of this book, Kristin put in countless hours reading and commenting on more recent versions of the manuscript, sparing me no criticism (I hope), and for that I am truly grateful.

I would like to thank the many friends and colleagues who helped and supported me in this process, in particular C. J. Pascoe. C. J. has read many drafts of this work from the earliest musings to the most recent chapters. Her insight and friendship have helped keep me grounded throughout this process. Many other friends and colleagues offered support and commentary at various stages of this process. I would like to thank Leslie Bell, Marianne Cooper, Meg Jay, Teresa Sharpe, Anna-Lisa Ulbrich, Heather Thompson, Mark Harris, Jennifer Sanchez, Claire Jeannette, Monica Andrade, Elsa Tranter, Linda Flory, Youyenn Teo, Kerry Woodward, and too many others to name.

I am also grateful to many other academic mentors at the University of California, Berkeley, and beyond. Dawne Moon and Barrie Thorne guided me through the early stages of this work and helped me form the methodological and theoretical foundation of the book. Adele Clarke at the University of California, San Francisco, again stepped in to help a Berkeley student seeking training in medical sociology. Lawrence Cohen offered thoughtful commentary and his expertise as a medical anthropologist. This project would not have been possible without each one's wisdom and intellectual stimulation. My colleagues at San Jose State University have supported this process in various ways, and I would like to thank Amy Leisenring, Carlos Garcia, Susan Murray, Wendy Ng, Scott Myers-Lipton, Peter Chua, Preston Rudy, Tim Hegstrom, and Sheila Bienenfield. In addition, I would like to thank the San Jose State University Department of Sociology; the San Jose State University College of Social Sciences; the California State University Research Foundation; the University of California, Berkeley, Department of Sociology; the Graduate Division of the University of California, Berkeley; and the University of California, Berkeley, Center for Working Families for various grants that have facilitated my progress on this work.

A special thank-you to the Bay Area fat community; the Bay Area Size Acceptance Think Tank has been a haven in the harsh world of obesity orthodoxy. The experience and expertise of those in the Health at Every Size and Fat Studies communities has helped me to work through my ideas and learn from the amazing scholarship and activism of so many dedicated and brilliant people. Special thanks to Deb Burgard, Esther Rothblum, Sondra Solovay, Shirley Sheffield, Marilyn Wann, and Pat Lyons for all their help, inspiration, and encouragement. Pattie Thomas, a brilliant sociologist in her own right, has been an editor/formatter extraordinaire and I thank her for her patience as well as her expertise.

My family has helped keep me grounded in this process, and my parents, Peter and Linda Boero, have offered much support (and child care), even as they probably wondered why it ever took anyone so long to write a book. My grandparents, brothers, and not-in-laws have been generous with their interest and support, and it saddens me that three grandparents, Lucille and George Boero and Joan Nelson, who saw me start this process, did not live to see me complete it. Although this research started well before they arrived on the scene, my children, Clarice and Jackson Gray-Boero, have motivated me to continue to think critically about bodies and health in new ways. I hope that they can live in a world where health and self-worth are not reducible to a single number. I thank Amy for her patience, her unflagging belief in this work, her in-depth comprehension of anxiety, and for many other things that don't need to be said here.

Many thanks to my editors at Rutgers—Peter Mickulas and Doreen Valentine—for their dedication and patience. I would also like to thank the anonymous reviewers for their insightful feedback. It takes a village to write a book, and never has there been a greater example than this one!

Killer Fat

Introduction

Weighty Matters

In a 2005 speech at the University of Texas, then U.S. surgeon general Richard H. Carmona stated, "Obesity is the terror within . . . [and] it is eroding our society." In the same speech, Carmona added that the "childhood obesity epidemic" in the United States will have dire consequences for the future workforce and military (University of Texas Health Science Center 2005). Carmona's statement is meant to scare people into taking obesity seriously, not simply as a social problem, but as a crisis and a threat to national security on par with terrorism.

Contrast the dire warnings of Carmona with those of Tina, a woman I interviewed ten months after she underwent gastric bypass surgery: "The doctors told me I needed to do this for my health. Well, maybe I am healthier now but I am more normal and, deep down, that is why I did this [had surgery], and that is why I dieted my whole life, to blend in, to be one of the crowd, you know?"

Tina's comments are not unique. In researching this book, I interviewed forty people actively pursuing weight loss and spent time in diet groups, twelve-step programs, and weight-loss surgery support groups. I was surprised that, in the midst of a health crisis as seemingly catastrophic as the obesity epidemic, people engaged in various weight-loss programs seemed relatively unmotivated by the specter of obesity or even by the risks of fatness to their own personal health. Rather, like Tina, most of the people to whom I spoke talked about a desire to lose weight to be normal, to be able to wear a smaller size, to blend in, and to avoid the

1

stigma and discrimination faced by fat people. This pattern held not only for people like Tina, who had undergone surgery in order to lose weight, but also for people engaged in less invasive weight-loss attempts.

In the last decade, obesity has come to be seen as more than a physical flaw, a disease, or evidence of a character defect, although it may still be viewed as all of these. Obesity has become an epidemic. According to Carmona and others, the obesity epidemic has the power to weaken the military, health, and economy of the most powerful nation in the world. The phrase "obesity epidemic," developed and popularized in the early 1990s, is now commonplace in media, medical, and health policy descriptions of the current prevalence of overweight in the United States (Boero 2007; Saguy, Gruys, and Gong 2010). Skyrocketing rates of obesity among all groups of Americans, in particular, children, the poor, and minorities, have become a major public health concern and a driving force behind social policy. Newspapers, television shows, and magazines are filled with discussions of the "expanding American waistline" and the health problems and risks associated therewith. Weight, once grist for daytime talk shows and popular magazines aimed primarily at women, is now national and even global news, and network and cable news shows regularly feature stories about the obesity crisis. In the midst of this panic, policy makers scramble to convey the seriousness of the problem and create policy to "contain" the epidemic. Pharmaceutical companies race to bring new drugs to the market, legislators vote to make the cost of diet programs like Jenny Craig and Weight Watchers tax deductible, and surgeons and obesity researchers lobby the government for research funding and to get weight-loss surgeries covered by Medicare, Medicaid, and private insurers. These efforts often have a punative aim. In many states, schools have begun to ban "junk food" and send home "obesity report cards" warning the parents of overweight children of the future health problems their children will face. First Lady Michelle Obama has made childhood obesity the centerpiece of her official agenda. Beginning in January of 2009, obese Alabama state workers were forced to pay an "obesity penalty" of twenty-five dollars a month; and, in light of ever increasing health-care costs in the United States, insurers and employers have or plan to implement incentives that would reward people for losing weight and penalize those who don't (Fernandez 2008).

Fat people have been blamed for everything, including the crisis in health care, higher gas and airline prices, and global warming. Americans have responded to this through a dramatic increase in their consumption of diet products and services and a greater willingness to undergo increasingly popular surgical procedures for weight loss. It is estimated that in the United States alone weight loss is a nearly $60 billion industry each year, and the growth of this industry shows no sign of slowing down (Marketdata Enterprises 2009). Yet, in spite of or, perhaps, in part, because of these increased expenditures on diets and various weight-loss interventions, rates of obesity have continued to rise in many groups and stagnate in others.

On one hand, the media, health policy experts, and doctors scramble to convince us that we are putting ourselves, our children, and our nation at risk. They tell us that obesity costs society hundreds of billions of dollars a year and that children alive today are the first generation in a hundred years expected to die earlier than their parents, mainly due to obesity. On the other hand, fat people engaged in these weight-loss efforts don't see their fatness as a public health crisis so much as they experience it as an impediment to social acceptance and economic stability. Although their willingness to undergo weight-loss surgeries indicates a tacit agreement with the framing of the problem by doctors and researchers, patients' assessments of their own motivations and experience do not match up with obesity claims-makers' argument that these procedures are a critical avenue to individual and public health. This chasm is the central focus of this book.

This book explores the contemporary American obesity epidemic. More specifically, it examines the gap between the public health crisis of the obesity epidemic and the personal concerns of fat people living in the context of that epidemic. I take a social constructionist approach to the obesity epidemic. I do not seek to document and describe the empirical reality of obesity, its causes, patterns, and cures. Rather, I explore the process by which obesity has come to be defined as a social problem, one of epidemic proportions, as well as the material and cultural consequences of this designation. Although not an exhaustive account of its history, I look at key moments in the obesity epidemic's construction with an eye to understanding the contradiction between the public health crisis and the distinctly individual responses to the epidemic.

Taking a social constructionist approach does not entail denying a rise in average weight of persons in the United States in recent years. The concern here is not whether particular health problems are truly associated with rising weights. I also do not purport to know why people have gotten fatter and what, if anything, should be done about it.[1] As a social scientist, what I do offer is a critical interrogation of contemporary panic about obesity through an analysis that links this panic to larger social, cultural, and economic trends. Other social scientists have also critiqued obesity panic in its various forms by tracing the emergence of the epidemic and the economic and political interests involved in its spread, usually using various forms of textual analysis. Yet in this book I link an interrogation of the construction of the epidemic to the lived experience of the epidemic by moving beyond text and using in-depth interviews and participant observation to explore people's motivations for weight loss and the meanings they make of the obesity epidemic.

Obesity as Postmodern Epidemic

Throughout this book I will argue that obesity is what I call a "postmodern epidemic." In the medical literature and popular imagination, an epidemic is the outbreak of a disease and has historically implied a contagious illness, for example, cholera, influenza, or measles. However, the term *epidemic* is increasingly applied to diseases that are not contagious, for example, breast cancer and heart disease. Yet, in a postmodern epidemic no discrete disease entity is required for a phenomena to be identified as epidemic. Some examples of postmodern epidemics that do lack a pathological basis include teenage pregnancy, gambling, and school violence. In the case of obesity, in spite of ongoing efforts to locate genes, chemicals, bacteria, or hormones responsible for making people fat, there is currently no known biological cause of obesity, yet most experts and the public accept the use of the term *epidemic* to describe its current prevalence.

These epidemics, like the obesity epidemic, rely on the application of medical frameworks to phenomenas that are not inherently medical in nature. In other words, postmodern epidemics involve the process that sociologists and others refer to as medicalization, the processes by which an ever wider range of human experiences comes to be defined, experienced, and treated as a medical condition (Conrad 2007; Conrad and Schneider 1992). Medicalization is not a zero-sum game, and some phenomena are more completely medicalized than others. For example, pregnancy has been more fully medicalized than alcoholism and various other addictions. Moreover, the degree to which something is medicalized can ebb and flow given a variety of social conditions (Conrad 2007). Scholars of medicalization have documented how Western societies have tried to apply the language and practice of medicine to a wide array of complex social problems. Yet a lack of connection with a known biological pathology makes the question of diagnostic categories potentially more fluid at the same time as it allows for diagnostic expansion and the inclusion of ever more individuals within these categories. This diagnostic fluidity has been central to the obesity epidemic as changing BMI (body mass index) categories have dramatically increased the numbers of overweight and obese people.

It follows from this that another feature of most postmodern epidemics is that medical interventions rarely result in lasting solutions. That these problems have been resistant to narrow biomedical interventions should be of no surprise as these phenomenas are not primarily biomedical in nature. In the case of obesity, the well-established failure rates of diets, the failure of the pharmaceutical industry to devise a successful weight-loss drug, and increasing rates of regain and complications among weight-loss surgery patients all speak to the intractability of obesity and its resistance to both medical and behavioral interventions. Interestingly, it is this high failure rate of weight-loss efforts without a concomitant critique of the social valuation of thinness that makes the diet industry so profitable. In short, repeat failures make for repeat customers.

Postmodern epidemics clearly foreground both the positive and negative aspects of medicalization. With respect to the former, two of the recognized benefits of medicalization are that, in theory, it exempts people from moral responsibility for their problems and allows people access to resources and interventions to treat these problems. A recognized downside to medicalization, its tendency to depoliticize and individualize social problems, belies their complexity and, in fact, may counteract the potential alleviating of individual blame (Conrad 2007; Zola 1972). As this tension relates to obesity, nowhere is this dual-edged sword more evident than in the experience of weight-loss surgery patients. Told by surgeons that their weight is a medical condition beyond their individual control, they come to see surgery as a valid option. However, when surgeries fail or patients regain lost weight, individual explanations for fatness are drawn on to explain these failures. All of these tensions and paradoxes will unfold in the following chapters as they relate to the obesity epidemic.

If medicalization literally means to make something medical, then it is important to ask who or what drives these processes. While early theorists focused on the role of doctors in medicalizing social phenomenas, more recent scholars have focused on the role played by the media, pharmaceutical, and medical device companies and even by patients themselves in driving the push to define more and more of social life in medical terms (Barker 2005; Clarke et al. 2003; Conrad 2007). This points to yet another key feature of postmodern epidemics, including the obesity epidemic, namely, that they incorporate elements of moral panics.

A moral panic occurs when a phenomenon, occurrence, individual, or group of people comes to be seen as a threat to social values and interests (Cohen 1972). Historical examples of moral panics include witch hunts and white slavery, both of which were manifestations of anxieties about changes or threats to the prevailing social and economic order of the day, whether that be the subordination of women or the decline of the institution of slavery. Contemporary examples include satanic ritual abuse and Internet predators, which manifest concern about the threat posed by youth, technology, and changes in the nuclear family structure. These panics are driven by a constellation of "moral entrepreneurs" who play a key role in defining the crisis through their interest-based claims-making. They are aided by the media that disseminate and reify this sense of moral panic and indignation (Cohen 1972; Showalter 1997).

In her recent work, Kathleen LeBesco (2010) illustrates how obesity embodies the characteristics of a moral panic set out by Stanley Cohen in the 1970s (Cohen 1972). Most significantly for this work, current discussions of obesity are characterized by concern over the purported dangers of fatness, hostility directed at fat people and the culture that supposedly makes them fat, consensus that there must be something done about obesity, and a fear of fatness that is disproportionate both to the risk of fatness itself and to the threat posed by other social problems. I would add to this that in the case of obesity, the threat of fatness portrayed in the media and by experts is far greater than that experienced by actual fat people.

Fatness and fat people have indeed come to be seen as a threat to social values and interests, and long-standing negative images of fat people have been employed and retooled to justify policies and interventions that are aimed at halting and repairing the "harm" they have done to society. Likewise, as I explore in the next two chapters, the obesity epidemic was made possible by various moral entrepreneurs and a media willing to spread and reinforce their claims.

In its ideal-typical form, a postmodern epidemic is one in which partially and unevenly medicalized phenomena lacking a clear pathological basis get cast in the language and anxiety of more traditional epidemics. This partial medicalization is then fueled by a sense of moral panic created by experts and spread through the media.

Fat in America

Much of the construction of the obesity epidemic relies on our historical understandings of fatness and fat people. In order to truly understand the current panic about obesity, it is important, first, to briefly trace the contours of the history of fat in America.

The discourses of fatness prevalent in a particular era can reveal much about the social, moral, and economic anxieties of the day, such as concern over the roles of women; the place of the medical profession; suspicions about immigrants, minorities, and the poor; and fears about sexuality, the vulnerability of children, economic stability, and public health. These anxieties and more can be seen in constructions of the contemporary obesity epidemic, but they can also be seen at different times in earlier understandings of body size.

The first American weight watchers were health reformers like the Rev. Sylvester Graham and his disciples (Schwartz 1986). In the 1830s, Graham began his crusade against gluttony and sexual excess, urging a return to a "simple" and "natural" diet of bland foods. For Graham and others like him, excesses in food and sex were forms of self-pollution born of civilization. In addition to a diet of bland foods, Graham's crusade for food purity and physical and spiritual health also hinged on the participation of women, particularly mothers. For Graham, the battle against excesses in food would be fought "within the home, at table, by women" (Jutel 2005; Lupton 1996; Schwartz 1986). Graham's focus on food simplicity and purity generally reflected the moral reformism of the time and the need to defeat the evil of gluttony.[2] Other religiously driven health reformers like John Harvey Kellogg took up Graham's focus on food purity and health and continued to tout a link between poor food quality, ill health, and weak moral fiber well into the twentieth century.

Beginning in the early twentieth century, the burgeoning American concern with weight control spread mainly through diet advice appearing in popular women's magazines (Schwartz 1986). Though women were the focus of this weight-loss advice, the idea of a muscular aesthetic for men and a general devaluation of any kind of fleshiness were gaining ground.[3] As with the previous period of moral reform, the target of this new trend toward slimness was white middle- and upper-class women. With the decline of the corset and the rise of the flapper in the 1920s, there also arose a valuing of "natural thinness." This aesthetic ushered in a new standard of beauty for women, and thinness became a necessary component of "boy catching" and marriageability. In addition, as agriculture and industrial food production expanded, thinness became desirable as the association of fatness with industrialism, wealth, and prosperity began to break down (Campos 2004; Farrell 2011; Oliver 2006; Sobal 1999).

Although prior to World War II some patent medicines and tonics for weight loss existed, it was after World War II that obesity became more fully medicalized (Sobal 1995). Building on a moral model of fatness and with an aesthetic of slimness already in place, a model in which obesity was designated as a disease to be treated through medical intervention began to emerge.

Jeffrey Sobal (1995) identifies a number of factors contributing to this medicalization, including the rising status of the medical profession in the postwar era, the creation of various medical specialities related to obesity, and, in particular, the surgical subspecialty of bariatrics and the increasing profitability of treating obesity. However, Sobal also notes that the inability of medicine to locate an isolable cause or effective treatment for obesity has allowed it to be taken up in multiple specialities. He suggests that the presence of multiple medical models of obesity has both advanced and constrained its medicalization by opening up obesity claims-making to a number of medical specialties, yet the existence of multiple framings also weakens the claims of any one group. Nevertheless, what all obesity claims-makers have in common is a view that obesity is a social problem, a real and persistent threat to society, and that obesity can and should be prevented and *cured.*

Medicalization is also advanced by the ability to easily measure and classify phenomena, and obesity is no exception. The medicalization of obesity hinged on the development of ideal height and weight charts by the Metropolitan Life Insurance Company (Met Life). Suspecting that weight might be one easily measured physical trait predictive of mortality, in the 1940s statisticians for the Met Life set about charting the death rates of its policy holders using a height-to-weight index (Oliver 2006; Sobal 1995). The table Met Life arrived at was based on the weight at which a person had the longest lifespan for a given height range. Of course, the tables were not based on a random sample of the U.S. population but on retrospective data from Met Life's customers, who were far more likely to be white, male, and middle class than the general population (Oliver 2006). Although they provided a quick and easily intelligible way of classifying people on the basis of weight for the purposes of assigning risk for the insurance industry, the tables also appealed to doctors and public health officials looking for more and easier ways to measure health. By the 1950s the Met Life height and weight tables had been institutionalized as *the* way to measure overweight (and underweight) and maintained this hegemony for several decades. Though the methods for measurement and classification of body weight have changed a great deal since the 1950s, the normative and scientific measurement of weight remains a permanent feature of discussions of weight and weight loss. With simple measurements for overweight in place, along with the linkage of overweight to cardiovascular disease, it was but a short leap to intensified medicalization of obesity.

The diagnostic expansion allowed by the insurance tables created a population in need of management, and the medical profession's linkage of obesity with cardiovascular disease in the 1970s solidified the idea that fatness was in need of medical intervention. Although doctors had long acknowledged the intractability of fatness, the association of fatness with the nation's number one cause of death set the stage for medical partnerships with government and increased funding for obesity research, which has only expanded in recent years (Oliver 2006; Sobal 1995).

Once medicalized, obesity acquired its own armamentarium of treatments. Early on, medical interventions were focused on drugs like amphetamines, diuretics, and laxatives, and these treatments were primarily aimed at white, middle-class women. More invasive treatments, like jaw wiring to restrict eating, also became routine by mid-century. By the 1970s, intestinal bypass surgeries had become a more common method to treat *extreme* cases of obesity.

A crucial turning point in the history of fat in America and, ultimately, in the obesity epidemic is the development and ascendancy of the BMI as the gold standard for the measurement and categorization of weight (Campos 2004; Gaesser 2002; Oliver 2006).[4] The BMI was originally created in the 1830s by Belgian astronomer Adolph Quetelet in an effort to apply laws of mathematical probability to humans. Quetelet did not consider it to be a measure of health, but rather a measure of averages that fit with the nineteenth- and early twentieth-century scientific interest in measurement in general. Quetelet never intended the BMI to measure individual or even social health (Oliver 2006). Despite its long history, the BMI did not gain dominance as a measure of excess weight until late in the twentieth century. Prior to that, the measurement and classification of ideal body weights was under the purview of the insurance industry and their height and weight tables. Like actuarial tables, the BMI was not intended to provide a measurement of health. However, given its scientific origins and an even more simplified classificatory scheme based on a single number, the BMI came to be seen by the public health community, the medical profession, and obesity researchers as a better fit than complex insurance tables as a measure of obesity.

According to the National Heart Lung and Blood Institute (NHLBI 2011), "Body mass index (BMI) is a measure of body fat based on height and weight that applies to both adult men and women." BMI does not actually measure body fat but rather the relationship between weight and height. Prior to 1998, "overweight" was considered to be a BMI greater than or equal to 27.8 in men and 27.0 for women. In 1998, the National Institutes of Health (NIH) made the decision to lower the BMI threshold for "overweight" to 25 and for "obesity" to a BMI greater than or equal to 30 for all people regardless of sex or body fat composition, thus greatly increasing the number of Americans falling into both categories of "overweight" and "obese." Some estimates suggest that this change caused more than thirty million Americans to move from normal to overweight overnight (Hubbard 2000). The BMI therefore creates a statistical norm for body weight that currently classifies over 60 percent of Americans as "abnormal" and in need of some form of intervention.

The power of the BMI and other measures of health cannot be underestimated. Indeed, much of the cultural authority of medicine hinges on the ability of doctors to classify and diagnose not only actual diseases, but also symptoms, syndromes, and, most significantly of late, risk (Barker 2005; Foucault 1994). What is most critical about the BMI is that it both holds the authority of science and is a tool that can be easily employed for self-diagnosis, thereby allowing people to calculate for themselves where they fit in the landscape of the obesity crisis. A testament to this is the omnipresent BMI calculator found on websites ranging from the NIH to Weight Watchers and the many pro-anorexia websites that have proliferated in recent years.

Though average weights among Americans do appear to be rising, the fact that 60 percent of Americans are overweight or obese is largely an artifact of the 1998 change in the BMI cutoffs for these categories. This kind of statistical adjustment is not unique to the BMI. Similar adjustments have been made for other measures from cholesterol to blood sugar and have also had the impact of branding more people as diseased or at risk for disease. Also common is that these shifts in measures may be noted by the media as they happen but are quickly forgotten as adjusted percentages of those afflicted and at risk become divorced from their roots in changing diagnostic boundaries.

The widespread acceptance of the BMI as *the* measure of obesity and overweight has not been without its critics, even within mainstream public health circles. And yet the index serves a need on the part of the public health community and groups professionalizing around the medicalization of weight, diet, and surgical programs for weight loss for a simple, "easily understood," and easily trackable measure of obesity. Its utility has quelled any significant public debate on what it actually is that the BMI measures and whether or not that has any real relationship to health.

In the public health literature and the media, the BMI has been set forth as the sine qua non for the existence of an epidemic. The BMI shapes health policy and attitudes across institutions and settings from schools to clinics and businesses and beyond. It allows for the identification and problematization of specific populations, especially African Americans, Hispanics, and children. Media and health policy reports act to convince the public at large that obesity is a danger to the physical, economic, and social health of the nation.

Despite, or perhaps because of, the hegemonic framing of obesity as an epidemic, there are alternative, though subordinated, models of weight and health that have emerged alongside rising panic about fatness. Perhaps the most powerful counter-discourse to that of the obesity epidemic comes from the Health at Every Size (HAES) movement.[5] The HAES movement emerged out of the size or fat acceptance movement and has been around for over twenty years, but it has gained renewed vigor in the face of the current epidemic. The HAES paradigm approaches wellness in a way that it is not focused on BMI, weight, or weight loss and embraces diversity in body size. The HAES paradigm recognizes the social determinants of health and advocates for access to quality, nondiscriminatory health care for all, as well as access to safe, enjoyable recreation, nutritious food, and leisure time. However, for reasons I explore at the end of this book, these alternative framings of obesity have had little success in altering the drumbeat of the obesity epidemic.

So, we have arrived at a situation where, even as obesity is incompletely medicalized, the existence and significance of an obesity epidemic is generally accepted. Part and parcel of this acceptance has been the taken-for-granted equation between obesity and ill health or risk of ill health. What allows for the incomplete medicalization of obesity and a rigid belief in its associated health risks to coexist is the existence of cultural and scientific "black boxes" that contain knowledge about the science of fatness and the lives and personalities of fat people. The knowledge these boxes hold has become taken for granted and is thus not open to question, and the shortcomings of each can be compensated for by the others. As I show in chapter 4, as medical interventions into obesity fail, it is often engrained cultural knowledge about fatness, and not science itself, that is drawn upon to explain this failure. It is through the complex interactions and mutual reinforcement of science and cultural truisms about fat people that obesity achieved and sustains its place as *the* American public health problem of the twenty-first century.

The Road Ahead

In an effort to understand the social construction of the epidemic and the experience of people living within it, the remainder of the book is divided into two themes. Chapters 1 and 2 describe the framing of rising average weights as epidemic by various moral entrepreneurs and communicated through the media. Chapters 3 and 4 focus on the lived experience of people, like Tina, who participate in weight-loss programs or seek surgical solutions to obesity in the context of the epidemic.

In chapter 1, I detail the development and debate over the *Healthy People* series. The *Healthy People* series was developed by the U.S. Department of Health and Human Services (DHHS) to prioritize and track the health challenges facing the nation. Debate over the the place of obesity in this series of reports elucidates the conflicts between various obesity claims-makers as the entrepreneurial efforts of two organizations, in particular, played out in conflict over the prominence of obesity in the report *Healthy People 2010*. While all players involved in creating the report agreed that obesity is a central public health issue, the process of arriving at the final version of *Healthy People 2010* not only points to a ratcheting up of concern over obesity, but also reveals an telling rift between public health officials and professional groups in which the moral panic surrounding the epidemic became increasingly driven by the latter.

As mentioned, the media are central to postmodern epidemics in general and the obesity epidemic in particular. This is the topic of chapter 2, in which I analyze over 750 articles on obesity appearing in the *New York Times* between 1990 and 2001. In this chapter I principally highlight the media as a tool for the spread and perpetuation of the obesity panic pushed by moral entrepreneurs.

In the second half of the book, I move away from textual analysis and turn to the lived experience of fat people trying to lose weight in the shadow of epidemic obesity. Using in-depth interviews with members of Overeaters Anonymous and Weight Watchers, as well as participant observation in meetings of both groups, I look at how these two programs incorporate expectations of what women's bodies *should* be like as well as expectations about what fat people *are* like. This is the project of chapter 3. It is a mistake, though, to simply view all nonmedical weight-loss programs as "diets" since each follows a very different philosophy based on differing understandings of the etiology of "overweight" and "obesity." This chapter explores why, though they are not the demographic target of the obesity epidemic, white, middle-class women frequent programs like Weight Watchers and what role, if any, social concern about obesity has played in their decision to do so.[6]

As corporate weight-loss groups and smaller nonprofit groups like Overeaters Anonymous maintain their popularity, there has been a startling rise in the appeal of bariatric or weight-loss surgeries as a technique of weight reduction and control. I explore the motivations of surgeons and patients, as well as their respective framings of the surgeries, through interviews with post-operative surgery patients; participant observation at informational meetings, support groups, and a surgery convention; and a close reading of literature on weight-loss surgery, as well as an analysis of representation of such surgeries in popular culture. In part, the successful framing of the obesity epidemic made bariatric surgery possible, and the existence of bariatric surgery makes the continuation of the epidemic possible. Following from this, weight-loss surgeons are both key beneficiaries of the epidemic and a driving force in its reproduction. This is the topic of chapter 4.

To be sure, given my own association with fat activism and a critical stance in relation to current obesity orthodoxy, I will likely be criticized for not taking this crisis seriously or for being a fat person (which I am) with a chip on her shoulder. But given the cavalcade of social policy surrounding obesity and the implications of this for the provision and distribution of health care, along with ongoing prejudice against fat people themselves, critical perspectives are necessary; and my own prior research experience, as well as my status as a fat woman, allowed me access to arenas in which I would have otherwise seemed out of place.

The most significant reasons to study the obesity epidemic actually have little to do with the lives of fat people in the most direct sense. The most important reason to study the obesity epidemic is because it provides a window into the construction of social problems, the construction of health and illness, and, in a larger sense, the construction of what is normal. All of this occurs in a historical moment when these issues are not fodder for mere intellectual debate but have consequences for all of us and for how we as a society attempt to negotiate the terrain of health, health care, and, indeed, citizenship in an era when social support for health continues to erode and inequality continues to grow.

1

Obesity as a "Leading Health Indicator"

Public Health, Moral Entrepreneurs, and a Confluence of Interests

In November of 2000, the U.S. Department of Health and Human Services (DHHS) published *Healthy People 2010*, the third report in the *Healthy People* series started in 1979. *Healthy People 2010* is not simply a report on public health priorities. It is, according to then U.S. surgeon general Dr. David Satcher, "an encyclopedic compilation of health improvement opportunities" (DHHS 2002, v). Including 467 objectives in twenty-eight priority areas, the report is more comprehensive than either of its predecessors. In spite of its breadth, what most sets *Healthy People 2010* apart from the two previous reports is its identification of the ten leading health indicators (LHIs) listed here.

- Physical activity
- Overweight and obesity
- Tobacco use
- Substance abuse
- Responsible sexual behavior
- Mental health
- Injury and violence
- Environmental quality
- Immunization
- Access to health care

According to the report, these ten LHIs are meant to "provide a snapshot of the health of the Nation" as well as "highlight major health priorities for the Nation and include the individual behaviors, physical and social environmental factors, and health system issues that affect the health of individuals and communities" (DHHS 2002, RG-1). Expanding on this, the DHHS website (2010) states, "The Leading Health Indicators are intended to motivate citizens and communities to take actions to improve the health of individuals, families, communities, and the Nation. The indicators can help us determine what each one of us can do and where we can best focus our energies—at home, in our communities, worksites, businesses, or States—to live better and longer."

At first glance these ten LHIs seem to be commonsense measures of health and priority areas for health improvement. But on closer examination these indicators help tell a story about the role moral entrepreneurs played in creating the obesity epidemic.

In this chapter I do two things. First, I analyze the initial three published *Healthy People* reports to show the emergence over time of obesity as a central public health concern. The increased attention and urgency surrounding overweight and obesity seen in the report *Healthy People 2010* dates the emergence of the current obesity epidemic to the mid to late 1990s (Saguy, Gruys, and Gong 2010). Second, and most significantly, I show that the inclusion of obesity and overweight as one of the ten LHIs in *Healthy People 2010* had less to do with scientific evidence than moral entrepreneurialism (Becker 1963).

Looking at the debate over what should be included as leading health indicators, I also consider how these indicators might have developed differently in different contexts. Many different groups with conflicting interests were a part of this debate. Understanding whose interests won out and why is important for understanding the conflicts and contradictions involved in the ongoing development of the obesity epidemic.

Healthy People

In 1979, the surgeon general of the United States and the U.S. Department of Health, Education, and Welfare (DHEW) issued a report entitled *Healthy People.*[1] This was the first national report on health promotion and disease prevention and, according to its foreword, it was intended to "encourage a second public health revolution in the history of the United States"

(DHEW 1979, vii). The document is remarkable, first and foremost, for shifting the focus of U.S. public health priorities from the curing of disease to the preventing of disease and ill-health.[2] The significance of this shift is noted in the report's foreword: "Let us make no mistake about the significance of this document; it represents an emerging consensus among scientists and the health community that the nation's health strategy must be dramatically recast to emphasize the prevention of disease" (vii).

The *Healthy People* report was designed to set ten-year health goals for the nation and set up systems to monitor progress toward those goals. The shift from cure to prevention emphasized in the report can be summed up by the three things Joseph A. Califano Jr., then secretary of DHEW, suggests that we have learned about the causes of "modern killers." First, "we are killing ourselves by our own careless habits." Second, "we are killing ourselves by carelessly polluting the environment." Finally, "we are killing ourselves by permitting harmful social conditions to persist—conditions like poverty, hunger and ignorance—which destroy health, especially for infants and children" (DHEW 1979, viii).

Califano seems to emphasize these three causes equally, yet in the very next sentence he seems to shift this balance toward individual behavior and personal responsibility: "You, the individual, can do more for your own health and well-being than any doctor, any hospital, and drug, any exotic medical device" (DHEW 1979, viii).

This shift in focus toward individual behaviors on the part of public health scholars and policy makers has been noted by others (Clarke et al. 2003; Conrad 1992) and is frequently dated to the 1970s and 1980s, placing *Healthy People* firmly at the front end of this trend. This first *Healthy People* report focused exclusively on prevention through the establishment of goals for health improvement in five life stages: infancy, childhood, adolescence, adulthood, and older age.

In the first *Healthy People*, "overweight" and "obesity" are only mentioned twice in the entire text, and the attention paid to excess weight takes up less than 2 full pages of text in the 177-page report.[3] The first mention appears in a section on childhood nutrition. According to the report, obesity often begins in childhood. Case in point, among adults who are obese, one-third are said to have been overweight as children.

By extension, therefore, priority must be placed on preventive measured directed toward children and adolescents.

The second time weight is discussed, it is in the context of nutrition and health promotion. In a half-page section devoted to "the obesity problem," the report cites the National Center for Health Statistics (NCHS), which found that among women ages forty-five to sixty-four, 35 percent who are poor and 29 percent with incomes above the poverty line are obese (DHEW 1979, 129). There is no information given as to how these rates were calculated; but, by whatever measure, obesity rates in men at the time of the report were low by current standards, 5 percent for men below the poverty line and 13 percent for those above it.[4]

In this first report, genetic or physiological causes of obesity are downplayed in favor of a behavioral model that locates the family as the primary factor in rising obesity rates. The report suggests that "a genetic component may be involved in obesity. But the social environment of the family—eating and exercise habits and a tendency to view food as a 'reward'—is one of great importance" (DHEW 1979, 129).

This statement implicitly puts the onus for childhood obesity on mothers, who are understood to be responsible for the development of their children's eating and exercise habits (Boero 2009). Consistent with the view of obesity that frames it as a problem of individual food and exercise choices related to early eating and activity patterns learned within the family, *Healthy People* offers as its only suggested solution to the obesity problem a laundry list of well-known behavioral techniques for weight loss. The report acknowledges, "There is no quick, easy solution to obesity; among adults it has proved very difficult to reverse on a lasting basis" (DHEW 1979, 129). Although the idea of reversing obesity has a clinical ring to it, the report also suggests that the most likely techniques to bring about weight loss are found in those who "inventory their food intake, avoid situations that would entice them to overeat, and gradually change their eating and exercise habits" (129).

The 1979 objectives represented a dramatic shift in the public health priorities of the nation yet were criticized for two main reasons: the lack of representation of the concerns of "special populations," especially racial and ethnic minorities and the elderly, and the lack of broad-based participation in deciding the issues and priorities for inclusion. According to the preface of *Healthy People 2000*, the second report in the *Healthy People* series, the first report was "viewed by many as a top-down, science-driven, professionally dominated set of objectives that gave too little weight to the social and quality-of-life concerns of people" (DHHS 1992, vii).

Healthy People 2000

Healthy People 2000 was published by the DHHS in 1990.[5] This report was intended to outline ten-year public health goals for the nation and to respond to the criticisms of the 1979 *Healthy People* report. In particular, *Healthy People 2000* appears to respond to criticisms that the first report was too top-down by placing an even greater emphasis on personal responsibility and behavioral change than its predecessor. Indicating a continuing shift in the meanings of health and illness, DHHS secretary Lewis W. Sullivan, in the foreword to *Healthy People 2000*, urges Americans to see health as a "positive concept," not simply as the absence of disease. He suggests that this process is already under way, and as Americans take a more active interest in their health, "they are coming to realize the influence that they, themselves, can have on their own health destinies and on the overall health status of the nation" (DHHS 1992). A focus on individual health behaviors is not only beneficial for the nation, it is empowering for individuals.

In response to the criticism that the 1979 report ignored the concerns of specific subgroups of the population, *Healthy People 2000* includes specific objectives for particular at-risk populations, including, for example, the poor and the elderly. However, it does not address previous concerns about addressing the health of racial and ethnic minorities or setting specific goals for these groups.[6]

In his preface to *Healthy People 2000*, Lawrence W. Green, D.P.H., a policy scholar at the Institute for Health Policy Studies at the University of California, San Francisco, suggests that, like the first report, the second report also places responsibility for health improvement on individuals. Green implies that this is understandable given the deep cuts the Reagan administration made in budgets for health services and health protection agencies, along with the simultaneous "development of policies of deregulation crippling the authority of health protection agencies" (DHHS 1992, ix).

In an effort to separate the objective health information contained in the report from a more subjective analysis of the political climate under which the report emerged, Green suggests that it is the political context and not the objectives themselves that aroused suspicion. He goes on to say that, in fact, the objectives in *Healthy People 2000* seek to "spread the responsibility" for public health among individuals, communities, and government. This theme of spreading responsibility over these three levels carries throughout *Healthy People 2000*, yet these levels are often given unequal weight, suggesting that individuals and local communities have as much power to improve public health as does the government, even in the face of ever-widening structural barriers to health care services.

The objectives and goals in *Healthy People 2000* are far more numerous and detailed than those in the original *Healthy People* report. *Healthy People 2000* contains 332 objectives organized into twenty-two priority areas, and the development of these objectives was based, in part, on comments from over ten thousand individuals and organizations. This increased public participation in the development of the 2000 goals was in large part a response to criticisms that the 1990 objectives represented the ideals and priorities of elites in the scientific community. One important effort to bring diverse groups into the process was the creation of the Healthy People Consortium in 1987. When the consortium was first created, it had 157 members, but by the late 1990s it had grown to over 350.[7]

The first sentence of the introduction to *Healthy People 2000* states, "In the last century we have learned that a fuller measure of health and a better quality of health is within our personal grasp" (DHHS 1992, 1). This is followed by a discussion of the leading lifestyle causes of "over 2.1 million deaths per year" (1): smoking, drug and alcohol abuse, inactivity, and poor nutrition. In *Healthy People 2000*, smoking holds its place as the number one concern of public health officials, and smoking prevention and cessation goals are prominent in the report.

The treatment of overweight and obesity in *Healthy People 2000* indicates that by its publication in 1990, weight had not yet gained the status of a major public health concern. *Healthy People 2000* does not include significantly more attention to overweight and obesity than the original *Healthy People* report ten years prior. Indeed, only 2 of the 332 objectives refer directly to overweight or obesity.[8] It is noteworthy that in *Healthy*

People 2000, concern about nutrition and exercise had not yet been collapsed into concerns about weight. The objectives relating to physical activity and nutrition are not framed in relation to weight-loss goals.

The terminology used to discuss weight in *Healthy People 2000* is also illustrative of an orientation to weight that did not yet view it as a national crisis. In the 2000 goals, the terms *overweight* and *obesity* are often used interchangeably and not necessarily in direct reference to specific BMI values. BMI values for obesity are not even specified.[9]

Moreover, the value of the BMI as *the* measure for overweight and obesity is actually called into question in the report, even as it relies on the measure when specifying weight-reduction goals. A footnote to one of the weight-loss objectives is of particular interest. It states that the use of the BMI as a measure for overweight is justified because it is easily and readily calculated using height and weight. The sense that the measurement is imperfect at best is captured in the following caveat: "Until a better measure of body fat is developed, BMI will be used as a statistically derived proxy measure for obesity" (DHHS 1992, 116). This, to some extent, is illustrative of a pre-epidemic skepticism about the risks of adopting overly simplistic criteria.

In the report, only two of twenty-one nutrition objectives explicitly address weight: "Reduce overweight to a prevalence of no more than 20 percent among people aged 20 or older and no more than 15 percent among adolescents ages 12–19. (Baseline: 26 percent for people aged 20–74 is 1974–1980, 24 percent for men, 27 percent for women; 15 percent for adolescents 12–19)" (DHHS 1992, 114) and "increase to at least 50 percent the proportion of overweight people aged 12 and older who have adopted sound dietary practices combined with regular physical activity to attain an appropriate body weight. (Baseline: 30 percent of overweight women and 25 percent of overweight men for people aged 18 and older in 1985)" (119).

The first of these objectives seems clear-cut. The phrasing of the second objective, however, is particularly interesting. Although overweight people are clearly seen as needing to lose weight, it is nonetheless acknowledged that there are people who are overweight, have sound dietary practices, and engage in regular physical activity. In addition, the objective suggests that children under age twelve should not attempt to lose weight. In sum, in 1990, overweight and obesity were seen as unhealthy and related to other public health concerns like inactivity and poor nutrition. They had not yet come to be seen, however, as the independent measures of individual and public health.

Healthy People 2010

The third in the series, *Healthy People 2010*, was published in 2000 and, as discussed above, included the ten LHIs. This is of great importance because the LHIs are intended to present a snapshot of the nation's health and health priorities.[10] While an entire section of the report is devoted to each of nine of the ten LHIs, obesity received only modest attention, subsumed as it was under the topic "Nutrition and Overweight." While there was a stand-alone chapter on tobacco use, for example, there were only three explicitly obesity-related objectives.

The three *Healthy People 2010* objectives that are explicitly related to obesity are as follows:[11]

1. Increase the proportion of adults who are at a healthy weight (DHHS 2002, 19.10).
2. Reduce the proportion of adults who are obese.
3. Reduce the proportion of children and adolescents who are overweight or obese (19.11).[12]

The first objective reported as a baseline that 42 percent of adults aged twenty years and older were at a healthy weight (defined as a body BMI equal to or greater than 18.5 and less than 25 in 1988 through 1994). The target goal was to increase this number to 60 percent. The second objective reported as a baseline that 23 percent of adults aged twenty years and older were identified as obese (defined as a BMI of 30 or more in 1988 through 1994). The target goal was to decrease this to 15 percent. The third objective reported as a baseline that 11 percent of children and adolescents between ages six to nineteen years of age were overweight or obese. The target goal was to decrease this to 5 percent (DHHS 2002, 19.13).

These three objectives do not appear to vary significantly from those presented in *Healthy People 2000* and are mainly concerned with bringing a larger percentage of people in line with current BMI recommendations.

In fact, these three objectives could be viewed as actually being less prescriptive than those in *Healthy People 2000*.

The most significant difference in the *Healthy People 2000* and *Healthy People 2010* report objectives is the change in baseline and target BMI values, indicating a greater reliance on the BMI as a measure of health. In 1998 the National Institutes of Health lowered the BMI cutoff for "overweight" to 25 and to 30 for "obese" for both men and women.[13] This increased reliance on the BMI happened in spite of the fact that *Healthy People 2000* had called for a more health-based measure of excess body fat than the simple height-to-weight ratio given by the BMI. However, no such measure had been adopted in the ten years between the publications of the two reports. *Healthy People 2010*, like the preceding report, maintains its utility based primarily on its easy calculability as well as its comprehensibility by the wider public.[14]

This acceptance of BMI as a scientific measure resulted in the diagnostic expansion of obesity. Even though average weights among Americans did rise significantly during the 1990s, the shift in BMI cutoff points had a staggering impact on the number of Americans placed in both categories, larger even than the impact of actual rising weight. As a result of this diagnostic expansion, the number of Americans classified as overweight exclusively on the basis of the 1998 revisions is over thirty million. It is this shift that made it possible to say that more than 50 percent of American adults are overweight or obese. Related to this, the 2000 report distinguishes between the categories "overweight" and "obese," whereas the first two reports had used these categories interchangeably.

Another significant difference between the second and third reports is the focus on children and weight. Earlier reports concentrated on childhood nutrition with only passing concern about weight. In the most recent report, children are seen as good candidates for weight-loss interventions, and concern over their weight is now central to concerns about weight in general.

Healthy People 2010 includes a long list of those diseases and disorders for which overweight and obese people are presumed to be at greater risk, including type-2 diabetes, coronary heart disease, sleep apnea, respiratory problems, and many types of cancer. The report suggests, "Maintenance of a healthy weight is a major goal in the effort to reduce the burden of illness and its consequent reduction in quality of life and life expectancy" (DHHS 2002, 19.14). Not only is this a matter of quality of life, it is also a matter of money. *Healthy People 2010* places a dollar value on the total costs (medical costs and lost productivity) attributable to obesity. Citing a study published in the journal *Obesity Research,* a publication of the North American Association for the Study of Obesity (NAASO), the report states that "total costs attributable to obesity alone amounted to an estimated $99 billion in 1995" (19.5).[15]

Given that, according to the DHHS, the list of diseases and disorders mentioned above are *related* and *associated* with obesity and overweight rather than *caused* by them, one would think that it would be extremely difficult to arrive at such a specific number; and to be sure, there is disagreement even within the obesity research community over exactly what that number should be and how it should be calculated. Yet, it is noteworthy that *Healthy People 2010* included such a number at all.

Healthy People 2010 presents a multifactorial picture of the causes of overweight and obesity, stating that "overweight and obesity are caused by many factors. These factors reflect the contributions of inherited, metabolic, behavioral, environmental, cultural, and socioeconomic components" (DHHS 2002, 19.15). Yet only nine pages earlier in the same chapter, the report asserts that "obesity results when a person eats more calories from food (energy) than he or she expends, for example, through physical activity" (19.4). It is this second and more commonsense model of obesity that appears to form the etiological underpinning of the recommendations given by DHHS for achieving the report's weight-loss goals.

For the first time in the *Healthy People* series, the discussion accompanying the weight-related objectives in *Healthy People 2010* suggests that doctors and other health-care professionals have a role to play in achieving these goals. The role of health professionals is to tell patients about the risks of being overweight and to give advice on behavioral changes thought to bring about weight loss: "A concerted public effort will be needed to prevent further increases of overweight and obesity. Health care providers, health plans, and managed care organizations need to be alert to the development of overweight and obesity in their clients and should provide information concerning the associated risks. These groups need to provide guidance to help consumers address this health problem. To lose

weight and keep it off, overweight persons will need long-term lifestyle
changes in dietary and physical activity patterns that they can easily incorporate into their lives" (DHHS 2002, 19.15).

Despite the clear assertion on the part of the DHHS that achieving
and maintaining of a healthy weight are key to the more general goals of
the report, like its predecessors, *Healthy People 2010* presents a vague yet
unambiguously individualistic prescription for action that is surprisingly
similar to that presented in the report published twenty years earlier. The
authority of medical practitioners is needed to impress upon patients the
seriousness of obesity and overweight, yet actual medical interventions
like weight-loss surgeries or drugs are not discussed or recommended.

Perspectives on overweight and obesity in the three *Healthy People*
reports remain consistent with a public health need to individualize
obesity in a way that skirts any discussion of social responsibility for
addressing structural factors known to be major contributors to disease
and disability. Over time, the reports increasingly frame obesity as a public health threat both as a risk factor and in and of itself (given its inclusion
as a LHI). Even as the crisis of obesity grows, the focus of intervention and
prevention recommendations remains firmly rooted in behavioral change,
nutrition education, and parental modeling of good nutrition practices.
While this micro-level and non-biomedical approach to obesity may have
served the needs of a government increasingly less willing to intervene in
questions of the structural inequalities of health, this approach did not
suit the needs of powerful and rapidly professionalizing *obesity-advocacy*
organizations and the mainstream obesity research community.

The Fight over Leading Health Indicators

To understand the disconnect between the public health and obesity
research communities, I turn to the development of the LHIs included in
Healthy People 2010. These indicators represent an attempt on the part of
the government to boil the nation's many health concerns down to a list
of ten that would serve to guide the development of public health policy
for the next decade. As we will see, these indicators clearly reveal the needs
of the public health establishment to simplify and individualize matters of
health and health care in the United States.

Those charged with the early development of the LHIs for *Healthy People 2010* were well aware that any set of indicators needed to be intelligible to the larger public as health issues, but they also needed to have political appeal, both for the purposes of the public health establishment and for those professional groups on whom DHHS relies to bring attention to the reports. It was clear from the beginning that the LHIs would not simply be a reflection of the objective health status of the United States but the result of a multilevel and complex interaction between the interests of a whole host of players. The case I present of the inclusion of obesity as a LHI is but one partial exploration of how these interests may coalesce in a given period.

The process that led to the development of the LHIs includes a series of reports. The first in the series was a DHHS report entitled *Leading Health Indicators for Healthy People 2010*. The report, put together by a group of twenty-two members representing several agencies within the DHHS, took on the following question: "Can a relatively small set of exemplary health indicators be identified which will reflect progress toward the health goals of the Nation—and do so in a manner which prompts public understanding and policy action related to the important determinants of that progress?" (DHHS 1998, 1.1).

To be sure, the question is largely rhetorical. The DHHS working group was formed precisely with the intention of identifying a small number of health indicators. Thus, a central goal of the working group was to formulate a short list of health objectives that would be meaningful to the broader public and "generate social and political interest" in meeting those objectives (DHHS 1998, 2.2).

The working group identified several limitations of the original *Healthy People* objectives that had undermined their effectiveness. These included, for example, the organization of objectives into five life stages and a lack of concrete data for tracking meaningful progress. The original report, so the working group concluded, failed to inspire national interest. The public was simply not interested in the life-stage health objectives, and even if they had been, there was no readily available way for individuals (or public health officials) to monitor success.[16] Any effective list of LHIs would have to garner political interest and generate public enthusiasm. The LHIs would need to "prompt both interest and action" for "strong-focused" interest groups to publicize the projects, arguably, to overtly politicize them in a way that a government agency alone could not (DHHS 1998, 1.3). The LHIs would then set the stage for working with the political and professional needs of these interest groups in future *Healthy People* reports and in the realm of health policy in general.

Rather than being organized by life stages, *Healthy People 2000* was organized into twenty-two priority areas that DHHS hoped would be seen as more relevant by lay and professional readers alike. The topical grouping of objectives had the potential to generate more political and professional interest than the previous age-based groupings, but the second report was slated to be significantly longer than the first. It would contain 319 health objectives. As such, "it became apparent that a smaller set of sentinel or key objectives would increase the usefulness of the document by serving as a focus of national attention and as a tool for monitoring America's health" (DHHS 1998, 1.3).

Forty-seven of the objectives in *Healthy People 2000* were identified by the DHHS working group as "sentinel objectives" that would be monitored in the future to assess the success of the report as a whole and would serve as priorities for the public. Even this effort to reduce and distill the objectives, however, was insufficient. There was still too much information to be easily communicated to the public and to capture public interest. To that end, the DHHS working group managed to identify eleven criteria to be used to generate a final list of leading health indicators (DHHS 1998, 1.3).

What can be gleaned from the working group's criteria is the need for the LHIs to be presented in compact and noncomplex form. After all, the criteria would be used in press releases, presented in print and visual media, and provided to patients in health-care delivery settings. In addition, having indicators that translated into obvious and effective policy action was essential. What was the point of the report if not to chart a clear policy agenda to improve the nation's health? Also on the minds of the working group was having indicators that could be readily measured and, therefore, easily tracked. As will be seen, this particular concern was influential in the final decision to include obesity among the leading health indictors and was a necessary step in the creation of the obesity epidemic itself.

The next stage in the process of formulating the LHIs is found in a series of reports created by the Institutes of Medicine Division of Health Promotion and Disease Prevention with the assistance of the above DHHS working group. These Institutes of Medicine (IOM) reports were presented to the secretary of DHHS in April 1999 (IOM 1999b, 1999a, 1998). This joint venture between the DHHS working group and the IOM committee started with the DHHS criteria. The agencies worked together to hammer out further details concerning how to best select the leading health indicators. In the end they agreed that the indictors should be worth measuring, measurable, intelligible to people who need to act, and capable of galvanizing effective action (IOM 1999b, 7).

One of the IOM reports noted that the indicators needed to be few in number and "be based on explicit models of health behavior and outcomes" (1998, 7). Like the DHHS report earlier, the joint reports with IOM show that the LHIs were primarily intended to address problems of individual and community behavior; and, by extension, policy intervention would facilitate this behavior change at the individual and community level. Rather than being primarily concerned with selecting indicators that would translate into significant health improvements as determined by biomedical evidence, the guiding criteria for selecting health indicators emphasized providing a set of measurements that could encourage and enable people to adjust their own health-related behaviors for the public good.

With the guidelines in place, then came the actual task of selecting the indicators themselves. Of course, selecting certain indicators for inclusion also involves excluding others. This was especially the case given the emphasis placed on keeping the final list of leading health indicators as short as possible.

One particularly interesting detail in this regard is the omission of poverty from the final list proposed by the IOM. In spite of the fact that the guiding criteria were largely oriented toward individual and community-level behavioral change, the IOM reports address *poverty* as an important indicator of health. In fact, the reported addressed a number of pathways by which poverty results in negative health outcomes (IOM 1999b, 1999a, 1998).

It is fair to say that, in terms of emphasis, the poverty-health relationship figures centrally in the IOM reports. For example, the following is from the final IOM report: "Committee members agreed unanimously that socioeconomic status and that poverty in particular are critical determinants of health and disparities in health behaviors and outcomes" (1999b, 71). Yet the report notes that the issue of poverty is "beyond the scope of the efforts of the U.S. Department of Health and Human Services" (71).

Although the report recognized the fundamental link between poverty and poor health outcomes, its omission from the leading health indicators "represented an awareness that social issues such as poverty are outside the purview of the public and private health communities" (IOM 1999b, 71). This is of great significance as it crystallizes a moment at which the LHIs could have addressed the many structural barriers to good health and did not.

So, if poverty, an indicator that appeared in all three proposed indicator sets, did not make it into the final set of LHIs for *Healthy People 2010*, how did it come to be that weight made the cut? This is especially noteworthy given the far greater emphasis placed on poverty in the IOM reports. In the end, the existence of the BMI allowed weight to stand out from any number of alternatives under consideration. Being overweight or obese became a leading health indicator in large part because the BMI makes these states easily measurable and understood. Overweight and obesity have also historically been seen as the results of individual behavior patterns, thus fitting with the individualistic approach of the *Healthy People* series as well as resonating with the long-established efforts of many Americans to lose weight through dieting. And, as I show below, there were powerful and interested parties heavily invested in seeing that overweight and obesity were included as indicators and figured prominently in the *Healthy People 2010* report as a whole.

Obesity as a Leading Health Indicator

In tracing the development of obesity as a LHI in *Healthy People 2010*, it quickly becomes clear that two organizations, the American Obesity Association (AOA) and the North American Association for the Study of Obesity (NAASO), were central in lobbying for its inclusion and account, in part, for a move away from structural factors in the LHIs.[17] The AOA, in particular, was at the forefront of making the case for including "overweight and obesity" as a LHI. Although these groups and the DHHS all favored framing obesity as a public health crisis, a divergence of interests between the AOA, NAASO, and the DHHS about the cause and cure of obesity accounts for it not receiving its own chapter, as was the case for the other nine LHIs.

On its former website, AOA described itself as the "leading organization for education and advocacy on obesity" and asserted that it was "the only obesity organization focused on changing public policy and perceptions about obesity. In only a few years we have become an authoritative source for policy makers, media, professionals and patients on the obesity epidemic."[18] Given the ever-expanding field of claims-makers about obesity, this was a remarkable assertion even in its early days. After its founding as a nonprofit corporation by two obesity researchers in 1995, the AOA became one of the most powerful and successful voices in lobbying for a disease model of obesity, including lobbying to secure government funding for obesity research and treatment. Members of the AOA included individuals, doctors, weight-loss clinics, and corporations.[19]

The AOA portrayed itself as being in a life-or-death struggle with the government, insurers, and others to have obesity taken seriously as an epidemic disease. In his welcome statement on the AOA website, for example, AOA president Richard L. Atkinson claimed that "obesity, the root cause of many health care problems, has been ignored by physicians, researchers, insurers, and governments at all levels."[20] The AOA described itself and other "like-minded organizations" as being the underdogs in a battle against a government unwilling to fully heed their warnings of the catastrophic consequences of not taking an epidemic like obesity seriously.

In response to this, the AOA's lobbying and advocacy efforts were primarily aimed at convincing the government to officially recognize obesity as a disease, getting more federal funding for obesity research, getting government programs like Medicare and Medicaid to pay for weight-loss surgeries, changing tax laws to make the costs of weight-loss programs like Jenny Craig and Weight Watchers tax deductible, and lobbying the insurance industry to cover weight-loss treatments and drugs. In all of these areas, they have been successful.

In advancing a disease model of obesity, the AOA positioned itself as a champion for the rights, health, and dignity of overweight and obese people. For example, AOA claimed that by identifying obesity as a disease, they were advocating for the destigmatization of the condition. Among other things this involved the recognition that individuals are not to blame for being overweight. Moreover, AOA boasted of working to change a culture that vilifies and discriminates against fat people, noting that discrimination against overweight people is "the last acceptable form of discrimination based on physical appearance"[21]

This appeal to end discrimination against fat people is a critical hallmark of the moral entrepreneurialism of the AOA. In claiming to champion the rights and humanity of fat people, the AOA set itself apart from the public health establishment. More specifically, the AOA argued that the public health mainstream reinforces negative stereotypes about fat people by approaching obesity as primarily a consequence of poor lifestyle choices. The AOA rightfully claimed that "discrimination against persons with obesity is rampant in education, employment and health care. Persons with obesity are daily offended by cruel jokes and insults."[22] However, the AOA's answer to the obesity crisis and the social discrimination faced by fat people was the recognition of obesity as a disease necessitating medical treatment. In the end, the AOA's campaign did nothing to dismantle the social and cultural norms and practices that disparage fatness and valorize thinness; fat people, not the social milieu, needed to be fixed.

NAASO described itself as "North America's leading scientific organization dedicated to developing, extending, and disseminating knowledge in the field of obesity."[23] Like the AOA, NAASO advocated and lobbied for increased funding for obesity treatment and research. But, unlike AOA, NAASO actually conducted and published research on obesity. NAASO members were almost exclusively research scientists and medical professionals. In 2004, NAASO reported that its membership included "1,700 basic and clinical researchers, who have published extensively, and care providers in obesity treatment and prevention."[24]

One of NAASO's primary activities was the publication of its journal *Obesity,* which it described as "the #1 scientific journal in obesity and the #2 peer-reviewed journal in nutrition and dietetics."[25] NAASO maintained a primarily scientific and professional membership by charging membership dues, which started at $200 a year for its most basic membership level. These fees, as well as the attendant level of membership benefits (that is, "basic" members were not allowed to vote within the organization, and those with more costly memberships were referred to as "fellows"), prohibited or discouraged less professionally invested members from joining. This, in turn, gave the organization a more exclusive membership base and greater professional legitimacy compared to AOA. In addition, NAASO required confirmation of professional credentials for any membership above the basic level.

NAASO adhered to a disease model of obesity and obesity treatment similar to that of the AOA. The groups shared a significant number of members. Whereas AOA often acted as the more political arm of the effort to professionalize obesity research and treatment, NAASO, situating itself as a more elite scientific organization, did not cast itself as having an overt political agenda.

The similarities and differences between AOA and NAASO played themselves out in the public debate over the content of *Healthy People 2010*. Both organizations recognized the importance of how obesity was addressed in a document as significant and authoritative as *Healthy People 2010*. Both organizations agreed that obesity had become an epidemic health concern and worried that the gravity of the situation had not been fully realized by DHHS. Both organizations relied on many of the same statistics concerning the prevalence, cost, and consequences of obesity. Despite these shared assumptions and concerns, the groups' strategies and tactics differed when it came to influencing the report's coverage of obesity. Still, both groups strongly advocated that *Healthy People 2010* present a disease model of obesity.

As members of the Healthy People Consortium, both the AOA and NAASO were part of a public debate on the content of *Healthy People 2010*. Both groups submitted letters to DHHS supporting the inclusion of obesity as a LHI, and representatives of both groups were present at public hearings throughout the development of *Healthy People 2010*. In a two-page letter to Surgeon General Satcher in 1998, NAASO voiced its support for including obesity as a LHI. Listing various diseases and conditions caused by and associated with obesity, as well as citing its measurability, widespread impact, and the presence of available data, NAASO also asserted that obesity meets all of the DHHS criteria for a LHI. Moreover, NAASO's letter noted, "Improvements have been realized in almost every health indicator outlined by Healthy People, with one important exception—obesity."[26]

Given this noted lack of progress, NAASO suggested that obesity should be emphasized in *Healthy People 2010* by making it a LHI and including a separate chapter on obesity. NAASO further specified that this chapter on obesity should be included in a section titled "Prevent and Reduce Diseases and Disorders." This last recommendation makes clear that NAASO took issue with the precedent established in the first two reports, wherein the content concerning weight was subsumed under the topics "Nutrition" and "Physical Activity."

The AOA also submitted a similar document to the DHHS and participated in regional and national meetings of the Healthy People Consortium. Where the AOA's involvement in the process was most evident was in its response to the draft of *Healthy People 2010* sent in late 1998 by the DHHS to consortium members for comments to be considered in the assembling of the final report. In the draft report, "obesity and overweight" were included as a LHI, but they were not given a separate chapter. Instead, the objectives related to obesity were subsumed under the focus area "Nutrition and Overweight." The AOA mounted a vigorous campaign to remedy what it saw as a "flawed design" vis-à-vis the placement of obesity in the draft document. More specifically, the AOA submitted a seventy-five-page document to the DHHS titled *Obesity: Increasing the Understanding of a Neglected Public Health Hazard* (1998).[27] In this document, the AOA provided a detailed justification both for keeping obesity as a LHI in the final *Healthy People 2010* report and for creating a stand-alone chapter on obesity, independent of the discussion on nutrition.

The massive AOA document opens as follows, "The United States is in the midst of an obesity epidemic contributing to the premature death, sickness, and suffering of millions of Americans. . . . Nevertheless, the *Draft Report of Healthy People 2010* fails to reflect the scale and impact of this epidemic" (1998). Indeed, throughout debates about *Healthy People 2010*, AOA and, to a lesser extent, NAASO positioned themselves as caring about a problem the government refused to take seriously. By claiming to be the only ones taking the crisis of obesity seriously, the AOA and NAASO bolstered their jurisdictional claim over obesity as well as positioning themselves on the moral high ground by urging a neglectful government to take the crisis seriously before it was too late (Abbott 1988).

The AOA took issue not only with the limited attention given to obesity in the draft of *Healthy People 2010*, but also with the implications of linking obesity to nutrition. This suggests, AOA stated, that obesity is "a voluntarily created condition by weak persons and therefore not worthy of the devotion of limited public health resources" (1998). The AOA noted that such thinking is "inconsistent with scientific understanding of obesity." AOA asserted that obesity is a complex disease with multiple causes, including many ill-understood biological and genetic factors.

Moreover, the AOA pointed out that even if obesity was given short shrift on grounds that it was a behavioral problem, DHHS had given other conditions caused by behavioral factors considerable attention in the draft. Diseases and conditions caused by individual behaviors, "such as smoking, HIV/AIDS, teen pregnancy, violence, substance abuse, and sexually transmitted diseases," were not downplayed in the draft (AOA 1998). At best, DHHS had been inconsistent with regard to how it presented so-called lifestyle diseases, and obesity was intentionally or unintentionally trivialized in the process.

The AOA response further speculated that the limited coverage of obesity in the *Healthy People* series reflects the mistaken idea that weight issues are adequately addressed by changes in nutrition and levels of physical activity. Thus, the report effectively minimizes the significance of obesity by framing it as a "transitional state between poor diet and real diseases" (AOA 1998).

The AOA report delineates four fundamental flaws in subsuming obesity and overweight into sections on nutrition and physical activity. First, according to the AOA, lack of physical activity and poor nutrition are only two of many causal factors for obesity. Second, the AOA states that obesity is a disease state in and of itself, not simply a risk factor for other diseases (that is, diabetes, heart disease, and cancer). The AOA cites other health organizations and agencies that also view obesity as a disease, like the World Health Organization (WHO), the National Institutes of Health (NIH), and the International Classification of Diseases. Likewise, the AOA argued that obesity is seen as a disease in much of the medical and scientific literature. Third, the AOA argued that focusing mainly on the three co-morbid conditions listed above ignores the fact that "there are 30 other major health concerns related or associated with obesity. . . . [T]reating three of more than 30 co-morbid conditions is unlikely to have a major effect in alleviating the significant mortality and suffering associated with obesity" (1998).[28] Finally, according to the AOA, the current DHHS strategies for dealing with obesity and overweight have failed to control them and their associated conditions. Citing the same lack of progress on the weight-related goals of *Healthy People 2000* that NAASO cited in its letter, the AOA contended that this situation is evidence that "clearly, a new strategy focused directly on obesity is needed" (1998). This claim by the AOA to have jurisdiction not only over the treatment of obesity itself but also over thirty or more co-morbid conditions via an obesity-centered approach furthers their claim to legitimate knowledge about most of the major diseases and conditions suffered by Americans (Abbott 1988).

The exhaustive efforts by the AOA, NAASO, and others to have a chapter devoted exclusively to obesity were in vain. In the final *Healthy People 2010* report, the coverage of overweight and obesity remained largely as it had in the draft document to which the AOA's seventy-five-page document had responded. In the end, the final *Healthy People 2010* report did include "obesity and overweight" as one of only ten LHIs, but in the report itself, discussion of obesity was subsumed within a chapter on nutrition and overweight, and its significance was undermined by listing only three obesity-specific objectives.

Upon the release of the final *Healthy People 2010* report, the AOA and NAASO responded quickly to what they saw as the continued and blatant neglect of the obesity epidemic by the DHHS. The AOA responded most rapidly and definitively to the report. On January 25, 2000, the AOA announced the release of a self-published document entitled *Healthy Weight 2010* as a direct response to the DHHS treatment of obesity in *Healthy People 2010*. A letter from then AOA executive director Morgan Downey to the surgeon general and secretary of Health and Human Services expressed his disagreement with the framing of obesity in *Healthy People 2010*. According to Downey, "Obesity is the most neglected public health crisis of the 21st Century. It is neglected not because many health leaders in both the public and private sector do not understand the importance of obesity, but because it receives a miniscule amount of attention and policy development at the federal, state or local level" (AOA 2000).

According to the AOA report, the government spends far too little time and money on obesity research and treatment. What is more, it spends no money at all on prevention. And yet "obesity is more intractable than cancer, heart disease, or smoking." Thus, the intent of *Healthy Weight 2010* is to provide "what *Healthy People 2010* does not: a framework for concrete action steps to improve research, expand education about obesity, institute prevention programs and include obesity treatment in public and private programs" (AOA 2000). The AOA's strategy to address its discontent with the final version of *Healthy People 2010* was to publish its own report using the language and style of *Healthy People* to claim jurisdiction over the diagnosis and treatment of obesity as well as to position itself and other obesity professionals as the only ones willing to take obesity seriously.

NAASO took a different approach. The organization teamed up with the National Heart Lung and Blood Institute (NHLBI) and produced a report entitled *The Practical Guide to the Identification, Evaluation, and Treatment of Overweight and Obesity in Adults*. The NAASO/NHLBI report was distributed directly to health care providers nationwide and endorsed by over forty organizations, including the AOA. The primary goal of the NAASO/NHLBI guide was to present recommendations directly to frontline health care workers. As noted earlier, it is in the interest of groups like NAASO to have other groups like the AOA do their financial lobbying while presenting themselves as disinterested scientific experts on obesity (Abbott 1988). According to NAASO and the NHLBI, "the Guide provides basic tools needed to assess and manage obesity and overweight. It includes practical information on dietary therapy, physical activity, and behavior therapy, while also providing guidance on the appropriate use of pharmacology and surgery as treatment options" (NHLBI 2000).

By teaming with NHLBI, NAASO worked within the public health community to counter the exclusively behavioral account of obesity in the *Healthy People* report. Through this alliance NAASO sought to interject a disease model of obesity into public health discourse and advance its own professional authority.

Although NAASO and AOA had slightly different responses to the DHHS's *Healthy People 2010*, both responses can be seen as indicative of moral entrepreneurialism. As moral entrepreneurs, AOA and NAASO worked to build their organizational power through claims-making about obesity, to discredit alternative framings of the issue, to influence other professionals dealing with obesity, and to convey the seriousness of the problem to the general public (Goode and Ben-Yehuda 1994).

Conclusion

The framing of obesity in the first three *Healthy People* reports differs from that advanced by professional groups like the AOA and NAASO. Whereas the former advance a behavioral model of obesity in which the most signifi-cant interventions are changes in individual habits, the latter adhere to and advance a disease model of obesity that requires biomedical interven-tion. In spite of promoting conflicting models of obesity and interventions, groups like the AOA, NAASO, and the government all have a stake in fram-ing obesity as an epidemic. This shared framing of obesity as epidemic in the face of huge rifts over the etiology and treatment of obesity indicates both the differing needs of the groups in question as well as the increased flexibility of the concept of an epidemic. All of these groups are served well by framing obesity as an epidemic. The DHHS portrays obesity as something of a *postmodern epidemic* in that it focuses on individual responsibility and risk (that is, as opposed to conventional epidemics caused by biological pathogens). In contrast, AOA and NAASO stake their professional identity and claims-making on a disease model of obesity, more in line with a conventional notion of an epidemic. Articulating the biomedical nature of the obesity epidemic is the crux of their moral entrepreneurialism.

In the end, the failure of *Healthy People 2010* to embrace a medical con-struction of obesity and emphasize it as a public health crisis opened a door for NAASO and AOA to assert their jurisdictional claim over obesity. As the leading public health agency in the United States, DHHS was not in a position to present a disease model of obesity in the *Healthy People* report. The agency sets public health priorities, which, it claims, can be dealt with by and large through individual behavioral change. Since its inception in 1979, the *Healthy People* series has emphasized prevention via individual behaviors. Thus, including obesity as a LHI is consistent with its long-standing agenda, whereas adopting a disease model of obesity is not.

In other words, the obesity epidemic itself emerged from a complicated series of moves and countermoves between various key players. The agreements and disagreements between these players came together to create the obesity epidemic as it is and precluded other possibilities. For example, neither a politicized framing of obesity that recognized its relationship to poverty nor a fully medicalized framing of obesity emerged, which allows us to see how it might have developed differently.

Of course, the debates and moral entrepreneurialism surrounding the *Healthy People* reports is only one piece in constructing obesity as a widespread epidemic. The claims of moral entrepreneurs must be disseminated to the public, and to a large extent the media are the vehicle for this expansion of expert debates into the public realm. In the next chapter I look to representations of obesity in the media during the same period in which the *Healthy People* reports were being written and debated.

2

All the News That's *Fat* to Print

The American Obesity Epidemic and the Media

Almost daily, newspaper headlines explore new facets of the obesity epidemic. New diet books and programs are promoted on the morning news and dramatic stories of surgical weight loss are staples of the talk-show scene. Popular magazines and websites span topics from entertainment to parenting feature stories about obesity, childhood obesity, and weight loss. The health-care reform debate is reduced to sound bites about obesity's being key to cost-cutting measures and to the funding of various reforms. More debate over President Barack Obama's nomination of Dr. Regina Benjamin for surgeon general centered around her girth than her qualifications for the position. Shows like *Honey, We're Killing the Kids, The Biggest Loser,* and *Celebrity Fit Club* have become mainstays of reality television. Discussions about more supposedly size-positive shows like *Drop Dead Diva* and *More to Love* include expressions of fears that anything that accepts larger people as normal will encourage further increases in weight and spread the obesity epidemic. The media attention given to obesity is unprecedented, constant, and central to the construction of obesity as one of the greatest social problems facing the United States and the world in the twenty-first century.

As we've seen in the last chapter, moral entrepreneurs are a necessary but insufficient piece of the rise of the obesity epidemic. The spread of postmodern epidemics as moral panics also depends on agents to disseminate the claims of these entrepreneurs. As scholars of moral panics have pointed out, the main avenue for this is the media, and the case of obesity is no exception (Cohen 1972; LeBesco 2010). The media, in all their various forms, are at the center of the obesity epidemic.

This chapter examines the role of the media in the obesity epidemic. I do this through a close analysis of articles published on obesity in the *New York Times,* the "paper of record" in the United States. The *Times* has been at the forefront of reporting on obesity, weight, and health since the early 1990s.[1] Between 1990 and 2001 the *Times* published 751 articles on obesity. In comparison, during the same period, the *Times* published 544 articles on smoking, 672 articles on the AIDS epidemic, and 531 articles on pollution.[2] In the broadest sense, these 751 articles are about obesity, fatness, and body size, yet these themes arise in a range of contexts. The sheer volume of media attention to obesity points to the fact that the obesity epidemic is not just a concern or product of discussions among policy makers and government officials. Indeed, this media dissemination of the *scientific facts* about weight and health reflects and reproduces what has become our larger *commonsense knowledge* about weight.

The amount of coverage itself is also part and parcel of the way the media spread moral panics and create a sense of urgency around various social problems. Many have analyzed how media overreporting on phenomena such as violent crime, child abduction, teenage pregnancy, and road rage has created a "culture of fear" and, in turn, contributes to ever-increasing media coverage of these issues to the effect that problems like poverty go underreported (Cohen 1972; Glassner 2000). Obesity is no exception and is perhaps the best example of the tenacity of this type of overreporting as the supposed epidemic nears the twenty-year mark with no abatement in coverage in sight.

The fear and panic characteristic of postmodern epidemics is reflected in the *Times* reporting on obesity since the early 1990s. In 1994, for example, the *Times* reported one researcher as saying, "We're frightened right now because obesity is an epidemic that has made all of us wake up" (Burros 1994b). The media, including the *Times,* present the obesity epidemic as a scientific fact. While a small percentage of the *Times* reporting on obesity does question some of the claims made about the link between weight and health, nowhere does the *Times* question the existence of the epidemic. The obesity epidemic has been portrayed by most media as a scientific reality. Even mainstream reports that question some received knowledge about fatness fall short of critically interrogating the very existence of the epidemic. Using the existence of the epidemic as a taken-for-granted starting point for reporting on obesity has the effect of silencing critical voices and training media focus on intervention and prevention of obesity, rather than on larger discussions about public health.

The limits on critical thought about obesity in the mainstream media are built on invisible but powerful *scientific black boxes* (Latour 1987). These black boxes encase issues that are considered to be accepted scientific wisdom and no longer open to debate. In the case of obesity, this includes knowledge of the general negative health consequences of overweight and obesity, the reliability of the body mass index (BMI) as a measure of health, and the general desirability of and positive health outcomes associated with weight loss.

Alongside and inseperable from the scientific black box of obesity, a *cultural black box* exists. In the media, preexisting yet largely unexamined long-standing fears about fatness, fat people, and fat bodies are deployed in the service of spreading moral panic. Taken-for-granted cultural assumptions about fat people—about what they eat, their emotional state, their lack of willpower, their laziness, and so on—serve as a powerful medium for the social acceptance of obesity as an epidemic. These cultural assumptions about fat people intersect with norms of gender, race, class, and sexuality. What we *know* about fat people is informed by what we know about minorities, women, and poor people. This knowledge is deeply intertwined with ideas about morality, health, and citizenship (LeBesco 2010; Farrell 2011; Metzl 2010). Thus, the scientific black box and the cultural black box of obesity leave little room for questioning the source of the moral panic and the basis of defining obesity as an epidemic. This comes through in an analysis of the *Times* coverage.

In 2000, the *Times* ran a series of fourteen articles entitled "The Fat Epidemic" in its science section.[3] This series featured articles written by some of the *Times*' most noted health and science writers, including multiple articles by Jane Brody and Gina Kolata, both of whom have written extensively on weight, health, and nutrition in the *Times* and beyond.[4] The series covers a wide variety of topics, including diet, exercise, weight-loss surgery, city planning, the genetics of weight, the diet industry, eating disorders, and childhood obesity, among others. The mere existence of the series sends a message of crisis and chaos, even as several of the articles in the series present ideas that can be seen as the beginnings of a larger-scale questioning of obesity orthodoxy.[5] From the articles in this series, along with other articles on obesity that appeared in the *Times* between 1990 and 2001, three themes emerge: chaos and containment, professionalization and common sense, and nature and culture. Taken together, these themes construct and disseminate the reality of epidemic obesity in a way that focuses on individual responsibility for health, confirms what we already think we know about fat people, and shifts attention away from structural determinants of health and well-being.

Chaos and Containment

In 1994, obesity researcher F. Xavier Pi Sunyer declared in an interview with the *Times*, "The proportion of the population that is obese is incredible. If this was about tuberculosis, it would be called an epidemic" (Burros 1994a). The obesity epidemic hinges on a sense that people and bodies are out of control in terms of their weight and that the consequences of this are both widespread and dire. A key moment in this rising sense of chaos was the 1994 release of a National Center for Health Statistics (NCHS) report that declared that, according to the BMI,[6] fully one-third of Americans were overweight or obese. In reporting this, the *New York Times* opined that "obesity has reached epidemic proportions in the U.S. and nobody knows quite what to do about it" (1994). An earlier NCHS study done in 1990 claimed that obesity cost the United States an estimated $69 million annually, and in recent years this number has only gone up (*New York Times* 1994).[7] Comparing the public health impact of obesity with that of cigarette smoking has turned into an important barometer of the epidemic with the declaration that "it won't be long before obesity surpasses cigarette smoking as the leading cause of death in this country" (Brody 1995). And in 1995, the *Times* reported, "Obesity *causes* 318,000 excess deaths a year" (Brody 1995). This estimate, too, has only risen in recent years.

This sense of chaos is furthered by the representation of obesity as a contagious disease that can strike suddenly and unexpectedly, threatening the physical and fiscal health of an entire nation. Food "basically runs riot through our lives" (Goode 2000), and extra vigilance is required to combat fatness: "families need to be more aware of where calories lurk" (Kolata 2000c). Fatness and calories lurk in the strangest of places; thus, common sense is not enough to tell us either who is fat or what contains fat. This assumption works to make obesity seem more like traditional epidemics of contagion. Sometimes overweight and obesity are self-evident; yet when trusting our eyes and experience, we may arrive at false and potentially dangerous negatives.

The propagation of fear of weight gain, reflected and reinforced in coverage of the epidemic, is continual. In an article on childhood obesity, written by Kolata for "The Fat Epidemic" series, the researchers she interviewed caution that you don't have to binge to get fat: "Researchers note that it takes just a tiny energy imbalance, a few more calories eaten than burned—for pounds to creep on" (Kolata 2000c). In an interview with obesity researcher Dr. Thomas Robinson in the same article, he states, "To gain 15 lbs. in a year, you only have to have an imbalance of 150 calories per day, which is one soft drink . . . [and] even a Lifesaver has 11 calories. An extra Lifesaver a day is an extra pound per year" (Kolata 2000c).

Real and potential victims of the obesity epidemic are not a circumscribed group; we all have to eat, and, therefore, we are all at risk and must be vigilant. In "The Fat Epidemic" series article on ethnicity and fatness, *Times* writer Natalie Angier reminds us that "the dread obesity epidemic that is everywhere in the news is not restricted to any race, creed, ethnicity, or slice of the socioeconomic supersized pie. As recent studies reveal, virtually every group known to demography is getting fatter" (2000). As these quotations illustrate, fear of fat is perpetuated by the idea that anyone can become fat at any time and with very little effort and that becoming fat is both outside of one's normal control yet also eminently within it—a national crisis with individual roots and solutions.

In the midst of this chaos and climate of fear there is little room for seemingly arcane debates that appear to derail the more urgent business of saving lives. This has the additional consequence of branding as heretical any individual or group that would step back and question the dire nature of the problem and the proposed solutions. Those who attempt to question the frenzy of the obesity epidemic or the relationship between weight and health are seen as not taking obesity seriously or refusing to yield to scientific reason.

Some of the most glaring examples of the failure to critically examine the epidemic came after the 1998 changes to the BMI categories for "overweight" and "obesity." In covering the story, the *Times* paid little attention to the fact that the largest recent increase in numbers of obese persons came in 1998 with the NIH's lowering of the BMI threshold for overweight. Overnight, more than thirty million additional Americans became fat when these revised categories were established as the reporting standard (*New York Times* 1998). Indeed, since 1998, many articles report that "more than half of all Americans are overweight, and 22 percent are heavy enough to qualify as obese" (Winter 2000), yet most fail to mention that the significant increase seen since 1998 is largely an artifact of the revised BMI guidelines, not an increase in people's actual body weight. This moment marks a missed opportunity to open the scientific black box of fatness by questioning the existence and severity of the epidemic.[8]

Creating a sense of chaos around obesity is a necessary step in the development of methods to contain the epidemic. Without a sense of chaos or urgency, it is difficult to reinforce the need for continued reliance on more familiar methods of weight loss, to say nothing of justifying more dramatic interventions that are both dangerous and expensive. A brief look at media characterizations of familiar interventions such as behavior modification and newer and more extreme methods like bariatric surgery shows how chaos and containment work together.

In the *Times'* description of behavioral approaches to weight loss and maintenance, only those who obsess over eating practices and display behaviors that, in another context, might be considered characteristic of eating disorders and food compulsions have even the slightest chance of avoiding becoming fat or maintaining moderate weight loss.[9] Obsessing about what and when to eat is cast as desirable, and the most dedicated dieters are represented as being "exquisitely aware of food, planning their eating and planning exercise to burn off calories and never letting a day go by when what to eat and how much to eat and how much to exercise is not on their minds" (Kolata 2000b). This quote points to the class-laden character of healthy eating as presented in the *Times* as well as how behaviors pathologized in the underweight are lauded in the overweight or obese (Boero and Pascoe forthcoming; Pascoe and Boero forthcoming).

Indeed, the success stories told in these articles reveal this middle-class bias. In an article on chronic dieting from "The Fat Epidemic" series, written by Kolata, all of the featured dieters are white, middle-class, thirty- to fifty-year-old women who have lost and kept off relatively small amounts of weight (twenty to thirty pounds) for a long period of time. Again, these women are lauded for having the characteristics of an eating disordered person. Women who count every calorie, exercise every day, and never "take a day off" are described as "skillful" and "dedicated," epitomizing the types of practices that could contain the epidemic if widely practiced (Kolata 2000b). In the context of the obesity epidemic, the need for this type of minute attention to food has extended beyond the world of women's magazines and into the mainstream of serious journalism.

Tellingly, the first article in "The Fat Epidemic" series is about gastric bypass surgery, the most dramatic biomedical intervention used in the epidemic (Grady 2000). There are several varieties of weight-loss surgeries, but all in some way involve sealing off or removing most of the stomach to limit food intake and bypassing parts of the intestines to prevent food absorption (Grady 2000). Designed to treat the most extreme cases of morbid obesity (BMI of 40 and above),[10] in the face of an epidemic, the surgeries are becoming more common. The American Society for Metabolic and Bariatric Surgery (ASMBS) estimated that in 2009 more than 220,000 of these surgeries were performed in the United States. This is up from 103,200 in 2003 and 40,000 in 2000. Over 85 percent of these surgeries were performed on women, and approximately 80 percent were paid for by private health insurers.[11] In other words, the willingness of insurers to cover the cost of these surgeries indicates an acceptance both of the seriousness of the obesity epidemic and of the potential efficacy of the surgeries as a containment strategy. This article presents cases of "people who had been massively overweight, had tried and failed at nearly every diet invented" (Grady 2000). Implied in this narrative is that, ideally, bodies and people would regulate themselves, but some bodies are so out of control that they need to be surgically altered to facilitate the kind of controlled eating that characterizes the dieting women above.

Alongside individual surgery narratives, the article gives statistics about rates, costs, and risks of obesity and cites widespread diet failure as a reason for such drastic measures. The article emphasizes the popularity and success of these surgeries, with only minor attention paid to their risks and costs. Given the seemingly magical potential of the procedures, the reader is led to assume that the benefits of surgeries outweigh the risks. The perceived chaos of the epidemic accounts for much of this lack of concern over the risks of bariatric surgery. Bariatric surgeries are framed as a "remedy of last resort" (Grady 2000), the most effective, if brutal, solution to the excesses of obesity.

The sense of chaos surrounding obesity fuels a drive to come up with new and increasingly invasive ways to contain, prevent, and cure obesity. This creation and spread of obesity panic is significant because it is a main avenue through which the claims of moral entrepreneurs like those in the Obesity Society are spread and reified.[12] This sense of chaos precludes debate as to whether the term *epidemic* is even the most fruitful or accurate way to describe the current prevalence of fatness in the United States. Therefore, a sense of chaos keeps the scientific and health claims of obesity scientists off the table, keeps them from being questioned and scrutinized in favor of a focus on intervention methods.

Professional Knowledge and Common Sense

In 1999, the *Times* featured an article under the headline "Scientists Unmask Diet Myth: Willpower." Quoted in the article is an obesity researcher who states that "the simplest and most judgmental explanation for the difference in behavior between [fat and thin people] is willpower. Some seem to have it but others do not, and the common wisdom is that they ought to get some" (Fritsch 1999). This headline and quote are emblematic of the second theme in the *Times* coverage of the epidemic: the conflation of professional knowledge and common sense. On one hand, the headline is meant to be a pithy commentary on how we really don't need experts to tell us how to lose weight; all it takes is self-control. On the other hand, the headline points to the phenomena of experts increasingly legitimating explanations for ill-health or risk using recourse to individual character qualities.

Since the early 1990s, there has been a remarkable increase in scientific and medical research on the causes and treatment of obesity. Reporting in the *Times* reflects this expansion. The obesity epidemic also presents opportunities for professionalization and profit that are reflected in the media. Obesity research, a former "scientific backwater" (Kolata 2000b), according to the *Times*, has quickly become a respected field. Genetic research into the causes of obesity has boomed, and research on viral or hormonal causes of obesity has been given much press. Yet even medical models of obesity draw heavily on individualistic theories of willpower and sensible eating. Even at the extremes of genetic or biological theories that assert that body size is largely predetermined, individual willpower remains the default explanation for obesity. A 1997 article about possible viral explanations for obesity illustrates this well as the final line reads: "Poor diet and lack of exercise are the overall main causes of obesity, doctors agree" (*New York Times* 1997).

The *Times'* coverage of two events, in particular, reflects the peculiar relationship between professional knowledge and common sense about obesity: the simultaneous release of the Institutes of Medicine (IOM) guidelines for the treatment of obesity and the launch of the Shape Up America program in 1994.[13]

On December 4, 1994, the IOM released a report entitled *Weighing the Options: Criteria for Evaluating Weight Management Programs.*[14] According to their website, the IOM is "an independent, nonprofit organization that works outside the government to provide unbiased and authoritative advice to decision makers and the public."[15] The report, distributed to all U.S. physicians, defined obesity as "an important, chronic, degenerative disease that debilitates individuals and kills prematurely."[16] The report recommended the increased pharmaceutical and surgical management of obesity. The *Times* called this report the first national "comprehensive guidelines for waging a successful war against the worsening epidemic of obesity" (*New York Times* 1994).

The day after the IOM report was issued, former surgeon general C. Everett Koop launched the Shape Up America program. Shape Up America was a "crusade to get the nation's weight down and activity level up" (Burros 1994b). The *Times* reported that Koop consciously planned the Shape Up America debut to coincide with the release of the IOM report only one day earlier (*New York Times* 1994).

Both of these programs were developed by credible scientists; measure the prevalence of obesity using the BMI; point to the economic costs of obesity; express concern about growing rates of obesity among minorities, children, and the poor; make recommendations for treating obesity; and legitimate their claims as scientific. Further, both cite the same dramatic statistics about public health costs and co-morbidity rates with other diseases. But, in fact, there is little agreement in the scientific assumptions behind the IOM report and the Shape Up America program.

Coverage of the IOM report emphasized obesity as a disease and focused on the potential benefits of drug therapies and surgery, yet Koop and Shape Up America viewed obesity as a problem of lifestyle to be dealt with through behavior modification. The *Times'* failure to note this divergence is significant. Scientific disagreement about the etiology and treatment of diseases and conditions is not unusual. What makes this situation worth noting is that the *Times* saw these reports as complimentary.

Amid the bombardment of scientific details on the obesity epidemic reported in the *Times,* the most scientifically committed researchers were still often quoted as saying that obesity is essentially a matter of diet, exercise, and willpower.[17] What is significant here is that while medical models are used to contrast with common sense or lay knowledge about health, in the case of obesity, these two seem to coexist peacefully in a manner that goes largely unnoticed.

A person looking to the media for information about weight, in general, and obesity, in particular, would be necessarily bewildered. There are almost as many theories about weight and weight loss as there are articles on obesity. On occasion, the *Times* acknowledges this confusion, even as much of the time its reporting seems to contribute to it. According to one article, in the midst of this epidemic, "people are confused" by the mixed messages they are receiving (Campos 2004, 45). Is obesity genetic? Are carbohydrates the enemy? What about fat and calories? Do drugs work? With so much confusion and lack of consensus about the causes of obesity and what we should do to prevent or treat it, the media as well as the scientific community often fall back on comfortable tropes about obesity that focus on individual behaviors.

The media's reliance on scientific measures of obesity has helped make this epidemic more closely resemble traditional epidemics. It also has the effect of professionalizing common sense. Theoretically, people could rely on visual cues or even numbers on a scale to know if they are fat, but in an epidemic more specific measures are required. Doctors also warn that you can't tell who is overweight by just looking at them, looks can be deceiving, and we need specific measures to tell us what our eyes can't (Kolata 2000b).

In the above article by Kolata, one dieter, Ms. Barton, takes solace in these measures. When she gets depressed about her weight she "goes to a website that gives body mass indices . . . and verifies that she is not even close to being too fat" (Kolata 2000b). Explicitly and implicitly, the *Times* reiterates to us that we must know our BMI, our body fat ratio, and the precise distribution of fat on our bodies to know if we are obese and to monitor our risk for obesity. In the article, a doctor suggests, "It is the responsibility of obesity researchers to tell the public that they really do have to think about food and exercise all the time" (Kolata 2000b). If obesity researchers need to spread the word about obesity, food, and exercise, the media are the channel they use to do it.

Obesity research and its presentation by the media both contribute to this professionalization of common sense. Overweight appears to have been medicalized in the course of this epidemic, yet at the same time common sense about eating and weight loss have become the default explanation for the obesity crisis. When doctors and scientists fall back on new incarnations of long-standing assumptions about willpower and individual behavior, they medicalize common sense. The extension of professional medical knowledge and expertise into previously non-medicalized arenas is a significant part of the medicalization process. Yet this professionalization of common sense is unlike past medical co-optations because it represents the professionalization of existing knowledge, not the replacement of traditional knowledges with medico-scientific expertise.[18] It is not just that new knowledge takes over, but that the old common sense is elevated and made scientific.

Nature and Culture

American consumer culture has become an obvious target in discussions of obesity. In a 1999 article, F. Xavier Pi Sunyer commented, "We live in a toxic environment with regard to obesity. Food is very palatable, very cheap, very easy to get. Labor-saving devices are everywhere. Everybody is working at desks, expending a lot less energy and eating a lot more" (quoted in Freudenheim 1999). Another article on childhood obesity suggests, "Pediatricians and Nutritionists say the reasons for children's expanding girth are not mysterious. They include a more sedentary life, with hours spent watching television, logging onto the computer, or playing Nintendo, which is coupled with a high-fat diet of processed food" (Lombardi 1997). Culture, in this case, refers to consumer and popular culture, especially its purported impact on children.

In tension with this indictment of culture is a belief in a natural weight and way of eating. This is drawing on a mythical past when, following our nature, we ate good food, not too much, and were not sedentary. This valorization of nature is seen in a 1994 article entitled "Truly Gross Economic Product," in which an obesity researcher suggests that "nature averts such portliness with the equivalent of a built-in thermostat that keeps the body at a more or less fixed weight" (Wade 1994). However, more often it is clear that culture has overrun our natural regulatory abilities. This statement suggests that nature regulates weight, but later in the article the same researcher tells us that, "unfortunately, its [nature's thermostat] settings are easily deranged by greed, genetics, and the influences of culture" (Wade 1994). The elevation of culture over nature as an explanation for obesity is the third theme found in the *Times* coverage of the epidemic.

Many of the *Times* articles on obesity portray nature as out of control and in need of harnessing, yet if nature is out of balance, it is culture that is to blame. Culture has made us fat. First and most prominent is the notion that something is wrong with American culture generally. Video games, fast food, television, lack of physical activity, supersized portions, and more are blamed for creating a situation in which people will "become as fat as their genes will allow."[19]

A culture of sloth and a sedentary lifestyle are especially to blame when looking for the origins of childhood obesity. Because children are constructed as more passive and vulnerable to the influences of advertising promoting sugary, processed foods, those aspects of American culture and personal behavior that are individualized in discussions of adult obesity are not so individualized in discussions of childhood obesity. Implicit in this critique of American culture is a blame placed on working mothers for children watching too much television, for children not having their eating habits more closely monitored, and for mothers relying on convenience foods for more meals. "In many households today, both parents work, so kids return to an empty house and settle in front of the television" (Williams 1990). This quote doesn't explicitly mention mothers, but, when "both parents work," it is mothers whose paid work is the cause of children being home alone. Families, in general, are often targets of blame in the obesity epidemic (Boero 2009; LeBesco 2010; Solovay 2000).

One article reports: "Experts say they are now beginning to realize what sociologists and family therapists have long understood: that just about everything begins at home—in this case, health and fitness. Unfortunately, many noted, they also appear to end there" (Williams 1990). Given their role as transmitters of culture, including eating habits, mothers come under fire from obesity researchers. As one researcher said, "If the child learns to eat from their overweight parent, who learned from their overweight parent, and Mom buys the same way and does the same thing she did years ago, and now that kid isn't even running and jumping the way kids used to, that child is in trouble" (Lombardi 1997).

Specific ethnic cultures are also targeted. As the following quote from an obesity researcher shows, the eating habits of other groups are not always seen in a negative light: "To see the national fat crisis in truly stark perspective, fly to Tokyo. . . . [T]he streets are thronged with slim, fit-looking people among whom the only corpulence belongs to American tourists or the occasional Japanese teenager who may have passed too often through the golden arches of Makudonarudos" (Wade 1994). Drawing on a crude version of the *Asian as model minority myth*, this quote suggests that in a culture that eats a more natural, traditional diet, what little fatness there is can be attributed to the encroachment of American culture. Though Asian cultures are lauded as having healthy eating habits,[20] Mexican American and African American cultures are constructed as the most problematic.

In one "The Fat Epidemic" series article entitled "Who Is Fat? It Depends on Culture," Angier (2000) notes that the high rates of obesity in African Americans and Mexican Americans are at least, in part, due to culture and also, in part, due to their overrepresentation among the poor. Researchers cited by Angier discuss the need for nutritional and health education among these groups. Those hoping to curb obesity in these populations also speak to the need to make fresh food more available in poor urban neighborhoods and make safe recreation more accessible. However, these researchers also report that it is hard to motivate black and Hispanic women to lose weight because these women seem less concerned with being thin than are white women. Dr. Marian L. Fitzgibbon, a professor of psychiatry and preventative medicine at Northwestern University, cited her own study that found that, in contrast to white women who begin to express body dissatisfaction at a BMI of 25 (the starting point for the overweight category), African American and Hispanic women did not start to show concern about their weight until they had reached a BMI of almost 30 (the lower border of the obesity category), independent of education level or social class. The higher levels of body satisfaction among of women of color are seen as a barrier to anti-obesity programs.

In an article on a California program to prevent childhood obesity, ethnic culture specifically emerges as culprit. This article, written by Kolata for "The Fat Epidemic" series, tells the story of Maria Sanchez and her children, participants in an experimental weight-loss program for Mexican American families at Stanford University. The article gives details on what the Sanchez family had been "doing wrong": "The Stanford program, which labels foods red, yellow, or green, with meanings like a traffic signal's, deems Pan Dulce to be red" (Kolata 2000c). Having discovered this, the Sanchez family switches from *pan dulce,* a sweet bread made from white flour and sugar, to whole grain cereal and nonfat milk for breakfast.

The problem of culture transcends individual households because these families also have to deal with other "social obstacles—like dinner at grandmother's house" (Kolata 2000c). Eating in extended families and community groups also runs counter to an idealized suburban meal, which is eaten at home and prepared by Mom and, therefore, is more tightly controlled. In this sense, culture is ethnic; and eating standardized, low and nonfat "green-light" foods prepared within the context of the American nuclear family comes to be seen as the natural and healthy way to eat. *Ethnic food* is an obstacle. Ethnicity is something to be overcome; reaching children and mothers first is the way to do it.

Thus, culture is a key point of intervention in this epidemic. This comes across clearly in an article detailing a program implemented in a small southern town by researchers from the University of Alabama.

Much like the urban program described by Kolata, this program targets African American culture in the rural South, an area in which a "culture of obesity" predates the Civil War and represents the most extreme contemporary example of "a nutritionist's bad dream" (Marcus 1998).

The town is described as one in which "there are three doctors, no hospitals, no ambulances, no 911 services. . . . The population is 79 percent African-American; the jobless rate is edging towards 14 percent and the median family income is $12,497" (Marcus 1998). However, according to the article, the *real* problem is to be found in local food markets, where all one need do to see the real downfall of this community is to "browse the shelves: along with ingredients for Southern staples like corn bread and fried chicken stretches a range of pig parts from head to foot, including brains and fatty ham hocks and tails. Pork chitterlings for frying are available in ten-pound buckets; fatback by the slab and fatty beef parts are popular, too. Lard flies off the shelves in eight-pound cans" (Marcus 1998).

According to the *Times,* program leaders are attempting to improve community health by "teaching women how to stay well by changing their behavior . . . and doing the unthinkable—banishing collard greens smothered in fatback and other traditional high-fat favorites in the rural South" (Marcus 1998). Again, women and mothers are targeted as an entry point into specific cultures as potential preventers of obesity. Program leaders suggest they are "building on community talent with women who are cooking for their children and passing on behaviors to their children and their children's children" (Marcus 1998). Thus, an analysis of macro-level social determinants of health is shunted aside in favor of a focus on *unhealthy* ethnic cultures.[21]

In the same article, the University of Alabama program centers on teaching southern women to adapt traditional recipes. The program and the article draw heavily on the language of southern religion and feature monthly community dinners of "born again soul-food" and "revered family recipes purged of their sins by two university nutritionists" (Marcus 1998). In a stark example of the continuing association of fat and food with morality and sin, before diners can eat their baked catfish and greens without pork fat, they have to "ponder the nutritionists' sermon on the evils of fat, sodium, and heaping helpings of sugar" (Marcus 1998). Again, not only are culture and its reproduction the problem, but *whitewashing* these cultures is seen as the solution. As others have pointed out (Mink 1995), food has long been part of the Americanizing process and has been part and parcel of naturalizing white culture as American culture. Ironically, returning to *whole, slow,* and *local* foods that resemble many of the traditional preparation and consumption practices scorned in the article has become a trend among upper-middle-class, educated, white *foodies.* Again, it is not so much the food itself that is marked as problematic, but those who are preparing and consuming it, as even lard appears to be making a comeback as a whole or even healthy food.

In blaming contemporary American culture, in general, and racial and ethnic minority culture, in particular, for the epidemic, there is an unspoken equation of nature with health. However, there is a wrinkle to this idealization of nature that is found in these articles. Sometimes, nature itself is problematic. As one researcher stated in the article on diet vigilance cited earlier, "if you leave it to nature, you are going to gain weight" (Kolata 2000b). These articles reveal an out-of-control nature that can't be trusted. Natural *drives, cravings,* and *urges* thwart efforts at long-term weight loss. Most of the articles about dieting and curbing desires for food orbit around case histories of women, indicating that it is women's nature, in particular, that is out of control.

Feminist scholars have noted that the linkage of women with nature derives from their reproductive capacity. By nature, women's bodies are unruly. Childbirth, pregnancy, menstruation, and menopause have all been used to justify women's oppression and the control and surveillance of women's bodies (Bordo 1993; Martin 1987). This long-standing ideological framing of women's unpredictable nature plays itself out in their presumed disordered eating. As others have shown, the control of these unruly bodies, desires, and appetites is central to dieting discourse (Bordo 1993). Women's association with children, nature, and the passing down of specific ethnic ways of eating coalesces to make women an easy and obvious target when culture is to blame for the obesity epidemic. Likewise, when nature is to blame for obesity, women's implicitly out-of-control nature is responsible. In short, at its most basic level, the obesity epidemic is about women. Thus, the media not only spread information about the epidemic, but also help fuel moral indignation about our toxic culture and the threat to public health posed by women, immigrants, and minorities.

Several stories in "The Fat Epidemic" series are notable in deviating from these three themes, particularly the theme of chaos and containment. One article takes on the marketing of fraudulent diet products (Winter 2000), and another article is about those who fight medical, employment, and social discrimination against fat people (Goldberg 2000). However, neither of these two articles questions the science or undesirability of fatness, even as the latter seeks to debunk some of the more common myths about fat people themselves. Only two articles in the series significantly question some of the received scientific knowledge about obesity, one article by Kolata entitled "How the Body Knows When to Gain or Lose" (2000a) and another by Brody entitled "Personal Health: Fat but Fit: A Myth about Obesity Is Slowly Being Debunked" (2000b).

In the first article, Kolata reports on findings connecting deficiencies in the hormone leptin with increasing weight. The article features an interview with Dr. Jeffrey Friedman, a researcher who does work on leptin and weight. Friedman suggests that it is a complex balance of genes, hormones, and brain signals that determine a person's weight range, not individual behaviors. Following from this, Friedman says that traditional diets are virtually doomed to failure because weight is largely outside of an individual's control.

Kolata also reports that these developments in the science of obesity have been of interest not only to overweight people tired of constantly failing at diets but also to pharmaceutical companies hoping these early discoveries might lead to blockbuster weight-loss drugs. Friedman and other obesity researchers quoted in the article adhere to a disease model of obesity and are optimistic about the development of medical interventions for obesity. Dr. Gregory Barsh, a Stanford University researcher, hopes to reframe obesity as a disease: "There's been a prejudice, a bias that obesity is a behavioral abnormality. . . . [S]omehow in the past, obesity was thought of as a poor relation to a real disease like heart disease or cancer. This misperception is being corrected" (Kolata 2000a). The idea of a genetic or hormonal basis to the epidemic is compelling in its potential to take the blame for fatness off of individuals and provide hope for a medical solution to the epidemic. However, these same medical theories justify interventions like weight-loss surgery; and, as I show in a later discussion of these surgeries, these medical theories are not necessarily incompatible with behavioral framings of fatness and often draw on the latter to explain the failings of medical science to solve the problem of obesity. Moreover, the article itself does not question the existence of the epidemic, dominant ideas about the relationship between weight and health, or the desirability and importance of weight loss.

In the second article, Brody presents the cases of several people who feel themselves to be both fat and fit, including Dr. Steven Blair, a fitness researcher at the Cooper Institute in Dallas. Blair and others have found that overweight and obese people who eat a low-fat diet and exercise increase their fitness levels and lower their risk for certain conditions even as they remain overweight. They have also found that fat and fit people have a lower death risk than thin people who are sedentary. This article stands out in the abundance of reporting on the dangers and costs of obesity for challenging the automatic association of fatness with lack of fitness and, conversely, the assumption that thin people are healthy regardless of fitness levels. Yet again, the article does not challenge the idea that, ultimately, being fat is bad and unhealthy. After telling the story of Cheryl Haworth, a three-hundred-pound Olympic weightlifter who can also do the splits, Brody cautions, "This does not mean it is O.K. to be overweight. A person who is lean and fit still does better in terms of health than someone who is fit but remains fat. But while everyone can't become lean, becoming fit is possible for anyone willing to make the effort" (2000b). Thus, thinness is still the gold standard of health, and obesity remains a threat to health even for those willing to take on the challenge of becoming fit.

Conclusion

The media are a critical part of the making of a moral panic and, in this case, the postmodern epidemic of obesity. Though the articles analyzed in this chapter chronicle only the first decade of the epidemic, it takes only a brief glance through more recent reporting to see that these three themes still remain the scaffolding of the obesity epidemic.[22] What is important about all three of these themes, and the way that they work together in the media, is that they construct obesity as a social problem of great urgency that is at the same time the province of experts yet also the responsibility of individuals and that targets both consumer culture and ethnic culture as the problem. What the interworking of these themes and general reporting on obesity have in common with the media spread of other moral panics is that the resulting panic or social problem diverts attention from more structural problems and posits individuals as both the cause and consequence of the panic (Cohen 1972; Glassner 2000; LeBesco 2010).

None of us has been spared exposure to the media drumbeat of epidemic obesity, but how it impacts individuals targeted by that panic is something that has been relatively unexplored. While individual cases may be presented in stories about surgeries, diet programs, or fitness regimens, little has been done to explore what undertaking these projects in the context of an epidemic means for the experience of individual people. Dieting and other weight-reduction strategies are nothing new; but when those efforts are seen as communicating something about a person's moral worth, do people's experiences of these common practices change? What about the experience of those who are engaging in new forms of weight control that only gained popularity because of the urgency surrounding the epidemic? In the next two chapters I turn away from the construction of the epidemic and move to the lived experience of those trying to lose weight in epidemic times. First, I turn to behavioral methods for weight loss, what most would call traditional dieting, to explore how the epidemic plays out in a context familiar to most dieters. Next, I turn to weight-loss surgery, a technique that has been around for almost thirty years but has gained popularity in recent years, probably due to an increased focus on the dangers of obesity and the efforts of moral entrepreneurs interested in advancing a medical paradigm of obesity.

3

Normative Pathology
and Unique Disease

Weight Watchers, Overeaters Anonymous, and
Behavioral Treatments for the Obesity Epidemic

The following vignettes come from my fieldwork in two of the best-known and most popular behavioral programs for weight loss, Weight Watchers and Overeaters Anonymous:

> Karen, today's leader, is tickled to show us her nametag because it has the autograph of Sarah, Duchess of York, on it.[1] She states giddily that she had "tea with the duchess" yesterday afternoon. She volunteered to check people in at an open meeting at a big grand ballroom downtown. She said the meeting was truly inspirational, that the duchess really got to the heart of her weight problem and was really open and honest. She tells how the duchess talked about the pain of being treated badly by the media and called the "Duchess of Pork," and how she was hurt by that and didn't want to live up to that name. The duchess would "smile in public and eat cookies behind closed doors." The leader then asks, "How many of you have done this?" Many hands go up, giggling shyly, and then the leader responds cheerily, "Well, then all of you are just like the duchess." (Field notes from Weight Watchers meeting, 2003)

The next person to share is Lindy, a thin/average-sized white woman who appears to be in her mid-thirties. She is still in her nurse's scrubs from work and is visibly distraught. She tells us she hasn't been to a meeting in quite some time and has recently broken her abstinence by eating something after 7 P.M. (she does

not tell us what, only that it was small and definitely did not constitute a binge). She feels intense shame at breaking her food plan and
the abstinence for which she has worked so hard. Yet, she adds, that
in some ways she is relieved because her break in abstinence has
shown her that she still has this disease, she is still a compulsive
overeater, and Overeaters Anonymous really is where she needs to be.
(Field notes from Overeaters Anonymous meeting, 2003)

If the obesity epidemic has been created and spread through public
policy and the media, the experience of living in an era of epidemic obesity
can be understood best through understanding what it is like to be overweight or obese and attempting to lose weight. The public health establishment has an interest in portraying obesity as largely the result of
behavioral factors such as overeating and underexercising, at the same
time as it supports the idea of an obesity epidemic. Following from this
individualized approach to weight taken by the Department of Health and
Human Services (DHHS) in the *Healthy People* series, the best interventions
into the obesity epidemic would seem to be those that work with individuals in an effort to change those behaviors that are making so many
Americans so fat. Here, I look at two programs that embody this focus on
behavioral change, though in strikingly different ways: Weight Watchers
and Overeaters Anonymous.

Much of feminist writing on the body, weight, and diet programs has
looked at how such programs both create and reflect unrealistic beauty
standards for women and reinforce normalizing pressures surrounding
women's bodies (Bordo 1993; Chernin 1994; Chrisler 1996; Stinson 2001).
Carol Spitzack (1990) says that in the act of dieting, women learn to inter-
nalize the male gaze and see themselves as an *other,* a project to be worked
on; and they build subjectivities based on what she calls the "confessing of
excess," a process she sees as central to weight-loss discourse. However,
Spitzack, like others who write about the connections between body size
and normative femininity, tends to homogenize all nonmedical weight-
loss programs together into the category "diets." While, undoubtedly,
some practices and assumptions thread through most, if not all, body
reduction programs, my research has shown that much is lost when one
fails to examine differences among programs.

As the vignettes show, and as I will elaborate throughout the chapter, Weight Watchers takes an approach to body reduction that I call the *normative pathology model*. Elaborating on the theoretical insights of scholars of women's health and bodies (Bordo 1993; Ferris 2003; Grosz 1994; Kirkland 2011; Laqueur 1992), I suggest that the relationship to food that is implicit in the Weight Watchers understanding of excess weight rests on the assumption that women, in general, are emotional eaters and, by nature, prone to excess. The Weight Watchers program relies on an understanding of normative femininity that meshes well with the knowledge contained in both the cultural and scientific black boxes of fatness so central to the epidemic. Thus, the seemingly vast differences between the average Weight Watchers member and British royalty are leveled by the experience of soothing hurt feelings with cookies.

The second vignette, from an Overeaters Anonymous meeting, shows an entirely different approach to food and eating. Lindy's experience of breaking her abstinence is not simply "cheating" on a diet; it is a serious reminder that she has a chronic and incurable disease that can only be managed through the fellowship of others who also suffer from the illness of compulsive overeating. I term this approach to food and weight issues the *unique disease model*, in which compulsive overeating is a disease, not the outcome of normal femininity, but an individual illness that is the product not of a culture of obesity but of characteristics unique to each sufferer. In this approach, excess weight is not the problem; it is but a symptom of the larger problem of compulsive overeating. In Overeaters Anonymous, fatness and compulsive eating are seen not as part and parcel of normal femininity, but as an indication of the compulsive overeater's inherent and incurable abnormality.

In this chapter I argue that an examination of specific behavioral weight-loss programs, rather than the category of "diets" as a whole, reveals that the discourses central to the construction of the obesity epidemic are also central to its treatment. I also argue that, as in the case of the media, public health, and medical constructions of the epidemic, women's bodies, women's roles, and women's mothering capacity lie at the heart of those treatments that line up most clearly with the individual/behavioral discourse of epidemic obesity.

It is a mistake to simply view all nonmedical weight-loss programs as diets. By separating out these two programs from each other, I show that while normative expectations of femininity are central to the definition of the problem as well as the identification of a solution for both groups, the techniques of normalization employed by both groups point to the complexity of defining oneself against a set of ever-shifting norms. I identify two very different approaches to weight taken by the two groups. Through the identification and analysis of these two approaches, I show how the question of whether or not it is a part of normal femininity for women to have a troubled relationship to food determines which techniques each group deems most effective. In other words, is pathology determined by expectations of femininity that posit women as irrational, over-emotional, excessive, and volatile, or is pathology determined against an understanding of an appropriate orientation to food and eating that hinges on supposedly universal norms of rationality, calculation, and detachment?

I also show that regardless of each group's particular perspective on the etiology of obesity, both the unique disease and normative pathology models allow for recourse to individual flaws to account for the failings of members. Thus, while all weight-loss programs may have the normalization of the body as their goal, not all are so focused on the normalizing of the self. This permanent abnormalcy of compulsive overeaters in part accounts for why Overeaters Anonymous is far less responsive than Weight Watchers to the language of the obesity epidemic.

In focusing on behavioral methods for weight loss, I am looking at those programs that encourage people to change their eating behaviors and ways of thinking about food rather than looking for biomedical treatments for overweight and obesity. As I discuss below, Weight Watchers and Overeaters Anonymous have significantly different frameworks for understanding behavioral changes as they relate to weight and weight loss and to the obesity epidemic. The former program embraces a behaviorism that much more closely approximates classic psychological understandings of behavior modification, while the latter takes a more addiction-based approach based on the twelve-step model.

Understanding the similarities and differences between these programs and participants in them can show how the designation of an obesity epidemic has affected or failed to affect people's motivation for weight loss, how they think about health, and how they understand the epidemic.

This chapter will also show how the programs themselves, both distinctly nonmedical in nature and philosophy, have negotiated the increasing focus on the relationship between weight and health. Both programs have in some way integrated the language of the obesity epidemic, but both do so in ways that do not compromise their original philosophies and methods, possibly pointing to the adaptability of the postmodern epidemic as a social form as well as the flexibility of disciplinary techniques in an era of normalization. Disciplinary projects like those of Overeaters Anonymous and Weight Watchers may share a common desire to normalize fat bodies, but they do not share the same concern with normalizing subjectivities. The discourse of fatness in Weight Watchers sees fatness as a predictable outcome of women's inherently disordered relationship to food, whereas Overeaters Anonymous sees fatness and food compulsion as the result of a disease with which only certain people are afflicted and which can never be cured but requires management through the achievement and maintenance of "abstinence" from problematic foods and behaviors. Weight Watchers encourages members to see themselves as normatively pathological, whereas Overeaters Anonymous members see themselves as chronically and incurably abnormal.

Weight Watchers

My first day at Weight Watchers! I walk in the door at 11:30 A.M. and get in line at the front desk, where two older women, whom I would later learn are volunteers, check me in. A gray-haired white woman, likely in her early sixties, welcomes me and goes over payment plans. I pay for my first week and registration fee and am given my weight booklet. While I am standing there, I buy a packet of the one-point Weight Watchers gummy candies that are displayed on the counter. The volunteer who is registering me tells me that every time I come to a meeting I will first go to the open, alphabetized files across from the registration desk, get my booklet, and take it with me to get weighed in the back. After weighing me, the weigher will refile it. They also give me a *Getting Started* booklet, explaining the way the point system works and containing an index with the point values of many common foods, and a food journal for the first week.[2] The receptionist then congratulates me on making such a positive step by joining Weight

Watchers and directs me to the back of the room, where a group of women wait to be weighed.

I walk around the meeting room before getting in the weigh-in line, looking at products and reading the posters that cover the walls. The meeting room is long and fairly narrow, with the registration area in front, the meeting area in the middle, and the weigh-in area toward the back. There are about fifty chairs arranged in three rows in front of a large white dry-eraser board. To the right of the board is a large bookshelf filled with Weight Watchers products like granola bars, sugar-free candies, shake mixes, scales, recipe books, mugs, and a few other things. During the meeting, Sharon, today's leader, refers us to a product that she and others had found to be particularly useful, a serving spoon that doubles as a portion control measure so that one can serve food and measure Weight Watchers serving sizes without anyone else having to know.

Pictures of food and their point values are everywhere. Food is a main topic in Weight Watchers. Bright posters on the wall give suggestions for what members can choose if they are looking for snacks and meals of varying point values. There are charts showing portions of various foods (actual size) and their corresponding point values and possible lower-point fast-food choices. Some of the women have already gathered in the meeting chairs and are leafing through one of the newer Weight Watchers cookbooks and discussing recipes and the different food products on the shelves.

A few more women come in as I look at the walls. I hear a yelp of joy from the scales. Later I find out that one of the women has met her goal for the second time (after a relapse years ago) and regained her status as a lifetime member.

I stand in line behind several women who are chatting animatedly, as are many of the other women in the room, creating an upbeat atmosphere, the mood I will consistently find during my weeks at Weight Watchers. While I am waiting my turn, I read a brightly colored display of "before" and "after" pictures and testimonials on the wall next to me. The testimonials are from people who have attended meetings at this location but are very similar to the ones on the Weight Watchers website and in the written materials. Most of them talk about traditional feminine concerns, like looking better and fitting into stylish clothes, but they also talk about things like health concerns, how weight loss helped these people lower blood pressure and sugar levels and generally feel better.

When my turn comes up, Sharon, also today's leader, leads me to an electronic scale in a small cubicle. There are four similar cubicles in a row, and, whereas people in line are talking in normal voices, people get quieter as they near the scales. At Weight Watchers weigh-ins are semiprivate with only the member and the staff member able to see the number on the scale. I start to step on the scale still wearing my shoes and jacket; yet, as I look around me, I notice other people taking off shoes, jackets, and even watches and rings with a curious automaticity before stepping on the scale. Most of the women use the bathroom before weighing, and many of my interviewees have told me that they wait until after being weighed to eat anything on weigh-in day.

The scale shows me at 222.8 pounds. Sharon then points to the Weight Watchers guide that shows that my goal weight should be between 116 and 140 pounds.[3] Sharon shows me where my chart will be stored and applauds me for joining at this time of year, saying that the holidays are a hard time to start a weight-loss program. She points out my daily point range (twenty-four to twenty-nine) in my *Getting Started* booklet and tells me she will talk to me and the other newcomers after the meeting and explain more. She concludes my weigh-in by handing me a new weekly recipe handout and saying that the key lime pie was really good. Sharon then says it is time for the meeting to begin and we all take our seats and focus on Sharon at the front of the room.

Weight Watchers has long been the benchmark of diet programs, with over 97 percent of American women recognizing the Weight Watchers name.[4] Yet its founder, Jean Nidetch, had anything but business in mind when she started holding meetings in the living room of her New Jersey apartment in 1961. In her book, *The Memoir of a Successful Loser: The Story of Weight Watchers* (1972), Nidetch chronicles her own lifelong struggle with weight. After many failed attempts at sustained weight loss, Nidetch found herself yet again determined to lose weight after an acquaintance she ran into at a supermarket mistook her for pregnant. As a last ditch effort, Nidetch found herself in the New York Department of Public Health Obesity Clinic. At the clinic she was given a very strict diet that she was told she had to follow to the letter. Though she was not hungry and consistently lost weight on the diet, Nidetch found herself "cheating" on her diet by hiding cookies in a bathroom laundry hamper and then eating them in the middle of the night. On weigh-in days at the clinic, she would lie about her midnight cookies to a clinic nurse who was suspicious of her when she continued to lose weight but not at the rate the clinic found acceptable. In Nidetch's words, "The problem was all the lying. I planned lies while I sat in the subway going to the clinic. I had to lie because I couldn't tell her (the nurse) about the cookies. Someone who had never been fat would never understand what I was going through" (1972, 68).

After this episode, Nidetch invited some friends over to talk about her diet, the cookies, and the guilt she felt when she lied about it. Nidetch decided that the key to being successful with dieting was talking honestly with others who understood the process and were going through it themselves: "I needed the girls. I needed to be able to tell them about my difficulties. . . . I've found that all overweight people have this tremendous desire to talk. Maybe we're all 'oral' types—we have to eat or talk. We have to talk about our problems and what we're trying to do about them. Other people aren't interested. Skinny people have so many other things to discuss and, if you persist, you're a bore" (1972, 70).[5]

For at least the first ten years of Weight Watchers, Nidetch continued to use the exact same diet she received at the obesity clinic as the basis of the Weight Watchers plan. Over the years and in response to changing social and nutritional trends, Weight Watchers has gone through several different food plans, all implicitly or explicitly based on a calories-in and calories-out model of weight reduction.[6] For Nidetch, what was truly unique about the group that first met in her living room and now meets in thirty countries was the element of talk, of talking compassionately and honestly about the process of weight loss, the struggles of dieting, and the celebration of successes. Nidetch found that essential to having this kind of group work was to have the group leaders also be Weight Watchers members who had lost weight and kept it off.[7]

In the over fifty years since Nidetch started talking with her friends about weight loss, Weight Watchers International has become the largest corporate diet program in the world. It has been publicly traded on the New York Stock Exchange since 2001. Some 1.5 million people in thirty countries attend one of forty-six thousand Weight Watchers meetings each week. Nonetheless, as my interviewees attest, people are still drawn to Weight Watchers for the kind of talk and support Nidetch suggested was so central to successful dieting over forty years ago. Maggie, one of my interviewees, encapsulates this well: "I go to the meetings and I really love listening to other people's little tips and tricks. Seeing people get those stupid awards like totally motivates me. There's a woman who has lost ninety pounds, and she probably has at least fifty pounds to go, but every Monday I go there and I look for her. I am just so inspired by this woman. So, I think I like the atmosphere of the group." As Maggie's remarks show, in spite of the phenomenal growth of Weight Watchers since its inception, its focus on group sharing and rewarding success still resonates with members today.

Weight Watchers has always emphasized that it is not a medical program. Early on Nidetch drew up an unofficial health waiver and had anyone who showed up for the meetings in her apartment sign it. Now, Weight Watchers is explicit in its literature and on its website that they are not a medical program and cannot give medical advice. Nonetheless, in a nod to the power of scientific legitimacy among dieters, Weight Watchers does emphasize in its literature and occasionally in meetings that the food plan has been developed by nutritionists and doctors to meet nutritional needs. Weight Watchers also suggests that new members consult their doctor before beginning the program and particularly encourages this among children, nursing mothers, and others who may have a preexisting medical condition; but according to my interviewees, very few actually do.

Beyond the legal aspects of these precautions, they also point to an explicit desire by Nidetch to make professional knowledge and expertise secondary to experience and lay knowledge in Weight Watchers. Nidetch illustrates this early in her memoir when she tells of her experience attending and speaking at seminars and conferences on obesity: "Some time ago I was invited to participate in a seminar on obesity at the Statler Hilton Hotel in New York City. I was the only layman invited. All the others were psychiatrists, psychologists, sociologists, doctors of every kind, and I was the only one who didn't have a bunch of initials like M.D. and Ph.D. to put after my name on the program. So I decided to give myself some. F.F.H. is what I chose: Jean Nidetch, F.F.H., is what I chose. It sounded good. And that's just what I am. A Formerly Fat Housewife" (1972, 11).

In establishing herself early on as an expert only because of her experience of being "a formerly fat housewife," Jean Nidetch gave Weight Watchers the "common touch" that is still sought out by Weight Watchers members who have grown weary of the advice of doctors and other professionals who, perhaps having never been fat themselves, can't really understand the multifaceted issue of weight loss. She also implicitly reinforced the notion that weight is a women's issue, a part of women's normal pathological relationship to food and emotion.

Weight Watchers may, in fact, be one of the earliest organizational responses to what Jeffery Sobal (1995) calls the "medicalization of obesity," which he dates to the 1950s and which revolved around the widespread prescribing of amphetamines for weight loss. Marie, a white woman in her fifties, says that her early use of diet drugs in her twenties was "successful" in that she lost weight, but she was "a neurotic mess and wouldn't eat for days." After the fen-phen scandals in the 1990s, Marie decided to stop "looking for a quick fix" and "do something that might last." She decided to join Weight Watchers.

At the time I observed, the Weight Watchers program was based on a point system in which members are allotted a certain number of points per day. Members are given a range of points and told that if they eat no more than the upper limit and no less than the lower limit, they will lose weight. Point values are determined using a formula based on the number of calories, fat grams, protein grams, and fiber grams in a given food. For example, a woman of any height with a starting weight of 180 pounds would be given a point range of twenty-two to twenty-seven points per day. To put this in perspective, a small apple has one point, 1 cup of cooked brown rice has four points, 1 cup of spaghetti with half a cup of marinara sauce has six points, and a small hot dog without a bun has five points. Remembering portion sizes is key to staying within one's point range, and the leaders frequently remind members of this. Marla, a leader, recounted with a tone of caution in her voice that she had been eating an apple every afternoon as a snack and that she had been counting it as one point in her journal. Out of curiosity, one day she put her apple on her Weight Watchers scale and found to her dismay that the apples she had been eating almost daily weighed closer to eight ounces, a large two-point apple, than the four-ounce one-point apple she had been recording in her journal.

She reminded us that no matter how long we had been in Weight Watchers, we still needed to be vigilant about portion sizes.

Weight Watchers has tried, with some success, according to my interviewees, to make the plan more flexible largely because it is no longer realistic to assume that the average member is a stay-at-home mom who cooks most of her meals at home. With the "Winning Points" plan, leaders emphasize that there is nothing that is forbidden on the plan, making it easier to stay on the plan while facing the challenges of eating in restaurants and at parties. While this is technically true, it would be difficult to eat a cheeseburger, which can, depending on the burger, eat up all of one's daily points, and still be able to get through the rest of the day without fasting. Indeed, according to the point values listed in the week-one booklet, one fast-food taco without sauce is fifteen points. Thus, one could arrange one's daily points to include a "treat," but this requires maneuvering one's remaining points to ensure that one could still eat three balanced meals in that day.

This formulaic structure carries over into Weight Watchers meetings as well. After a half-hour period for weigh-ins, the meetings are always thirty minutes in length and are lead by a paid Weight Watchers "lifetime member."[8] In the course of my twelve weeks at Weight Watchers, I observed four different leaders. All four were white women who looked to be in their forties and fifties and had maintained weight losses of varying amounts (between twenty and fifty pounds) for at least one year. Each added her own style to the meetings, but all followed the Weight Watchers meeting guide in the lesson portion of the meeting. During the time period observed, the leaders would cycle through a series of meeting topics each twelve weeks.[9]

The first five or ten minutes of each meeting are devoted to open discussion and the handing out of weight-loss awards. After weigh-in, the weigh-in staff notifies leaders when a member has hit a five-pound marker or has made goal, and the leader announces this during the meeting and asks the "losers" how they did it. In this part of the meetings, members share tips, ask questions, and discuss difficulties. Members often express surprise at just how much or little one cup or three ounces of a given food are, or they ask other members questions about their journaling strategies. Weighing and measuring and the importance of portion control are often central to the questions and comments during this period. Invariably, leaders take up the topic of portion sizes and remind members that one of the greatest mistakes people make on the Weight Watchers plan is thinking that they can "eyeball" portion sizes.[10] Members are encouraged to weigh and measure their food using a Weight Watchers scale, available for sale at the meeting. Members are also told they can purchase a set of serving spoons that serve exactly one cup and half cup portions, useful for foods such as rice; and, as leaders often point out, items such as these spoons can be used at the table with family and friends without anyone ever having to know that you are measuring your food right there in front of them. Following the Weight Watchers program yet not appearing to be on a diet is a frequent discussion at meetings.

Meeting topics reflect an understanding of the typical Weight Watchers member as most likely to be a white, heterosexual, and middle-class woman with children living at home. One day the meeting topic was positive thinking, and Marla reminded us that positive thinking is central to success on the Weight Watchers program. Another leader once urged us to not think "I have to drive the kids to practice" but "I get to drive the kids to practice." Around the holidays, meetings weren't very well attended, and one leader suggested it was because people were home with kids who were off school on break. This illustrates not only the gendered nature of assumptions made by Weight Watchers leaders, but also the implicitly middle-class focus of the program. Regardless of the specific demographics of the meetings I observed, the program most often seems to be geared toward middle-class women with children.

Men are rare at Weight Watchers meetings, and when they do come they are most often with their wives. At one meeting we met Jeff and Stacy, a young, white, married couple who had been on the program for three years and had lost over one hundred pounds together. Leigh-Ann, that day's leader, introduced them to us as two of her most successful members. Stacy told us that it was Jeff's idea to join Weight Watchers. In response to this, some of the women in the room clapped, others laughed, presumably at the novelty of a man being the one to initiate the couples' participation in Weight Watchers. Stacy told us that one of the best benefits was that, though she didn't know how to cook when she first got married, she learned to cook through Weight Watchers, and now she cooks

Weight Watchers meals for both of them. Other men who came to Weight Watchers often weighed in and left before the actual meeting started; one of my male interviewees suggested that this was because men felt the meeting topics were not relevant to them. Indeed, men's weight problems are often seen as the result of just liking to eat a lot, whereas women's are seen as a result of an inappropriate and emotional response to food. Men, then, often seek the structure of Weight Watchers—the weigh-ins, the food plan—but do not feel they need the mutual-support aspect of the program.

Like many programs that used to be called diets, Weight Watchers now calls itself a "lifestyle program." With increasing publicity about the overwhelming failure of diets to produce long-term weight loss, as well as studies about the possible ill health effects of "yo-yo dieting," nonmedical weight-loss programs have tried to make their programs more "livable" and maintainable. In order to do this, programs focused information about their plans on the variety of foods permissible, ease of recipe or prepared food preparation, rejection of a "crash-diet mentality," and encouragement of long-term success (Chapman 1999; Stinson 2001). Weight Watchers, in particular, points out that you do not need (though you may choose) to purchase any special foods to participate in the program. They also encourage "balanced nutrition" by suggesting a minimum number of servings of dairy, fruits, and vegetables, as well as by encouraging the consumption of water and moderate exercise.[11] Weight Watchers also encourages maintenance by offering free lifetime membership to members who have achieved their goal weight and continue to maintain it within two pounds up or down.[12]

However, according to most of the Weight Watchers members I interviewed, a diet by any other name is still a diet. Janice, a thirty-year-old, first-time Weight Watchers member, told me, "Well, they call it a 'lifestyle change,' but these days they really have to do it because the word 'diet' has so many negative connotations." Most made this assessment based on their perception of the central features of diets, writing food down, eating less, exercising more, weighing in, counting calories, goal weights, eating special foods, measuring food, an so on, and comparing those features with what they found in Weight Watchers. Three of the older women I spoke with were more adamant that Weight Watchers is, indeed, a lifestyle change. Annie, a fifty-eight-year-old white woman, told me, "[Weight

Watchers] teaches you how to eat normally; that's what I really need, not a quick fix."

This generational difference may be accounted for in part by the greater experience of interviewees over the age of fifty with "fad" or "crash" diets. All three older women had taken some form of prescription amphetamine in their attempts to lose weight, and all had done some form of liquid diet, fasting diet, or diet that involved eating only one or two different foods for an extended period of time. The younger women certainly had dieting experience and most had been concerned about their weight since adolescence, but most had not gone to the extremes the older women had. It is plausible that for people more accustomed to fad diets, the Weight Watchers plan would, indeed, be experienced as more of a lifestyle change than a diet.

In the logic of leaders, because it is a lifestyle change, people do not "fail" in Weight Watchers like they often do with diets. According to one leader, "in Weight Watchers, we are about feedback, not about failure. Through our *slips* we learn about ourselves and our eating habits and we have the opportunity to get right back on track."

On the other hand, the focus on "feedback, not failure" could also be seen in a more Foucauldian light; they don't fail because the prize of normalcy is always just ahead of them. In a program where a food journal can "be your best friend" and "self-monitoring is the greatest predictor of success," when they don't employ these techniques to their fullest, they need "feedback," not punishment (Spitzack 1990).

Central to this feedback is one of the key features of the Weight Watchers program, journaling. At one meeting I attended, the week's topic was journaling, and the leader, Leigh-Ann, reminded us that "journaling is the single greatest predictor of success in Weight Watchers." As a part of this topic, the leader wrote "tools for success" on the dry-erase board at the front of the room. The list read as follows:

- Journal
- Journal Diary
- Electronic Points Finder
- Etools (the pay portion of the Weight Watchers website)
- Points Bracelet

Leigh-Ann told us that all of these tools could help us to journal more accurately and efficiently, thereby contributing to our success in the program.

Weight Watchers has no formal sponsor system, but people are encouraged to buddy up and journal together. Journaling is a central component of Weight Watchers success; leaders remind us that people who keep a detailed point journal tend to lose more weight. When asked, my interviewees agreed with this statement. The journals themselves are very simple, folded paper booklets that are given out every week, with spaces to record what, when, and how much you ate and how many points each of those things contained. There are spaces to check off how many glasses of water and servings of dairy one has had as well. There is very little space for anything but an eating record on the free journals, but Weight Watchers also sells a journal diary with extra pages for members to record their thoughts and feelings when they eat or any food issues they are having. None of the members I interviewed used this more-detailed journal, and though many of them said they were lax in their actual journaling habits, all of them agreed that journaling is important, and most found that the more accurately they journaled, the more weight they lost. Maggie told me that she had this week's *group journal* and that it was making her realize that she was eating more when she stopped journaling than when she was more diligent.[13]

> Journaling totally helped me early on. I mean, just learning, like I memorized a lot of the point values of different foods and the whole weighing and measuring things. There are certain things you can kind of figure out even if you don't calculate the point value of a food, just by looking at a label, so that helped. That stuff actually helped a lot. I actually have the group journal; we do a group journal and I'm doing it right now for our group, so I'm writing everything down. I haven't journaled in a long time and I'm eating way over my points.

The reason Weight Watchers is so committed to the idea of journaling is intricately connected to its understanding of why people are overweight or obese in the first place. In Weight Watchers people aren't fat because they are genetically predisposed or because they have any kind of chemical imbalance that affects the way they metabolize food. People are fat because of bad habits. They don't know what is in their food, they eat huge portions, they eat for emotional reasons, and they don't get enough exercise. Because women are predisposed to emotional or disordered eating, monitoring exactly what goes in is critical if one is to lose weight. Women eat for often irrational and emotional reasons; thus, journaling is part of rationalizing that process and creating a way to go back and reflect on it.

Overeaters Anonymous

I had been meaning to go to this meeting for a long time. I was told it would be a "good one" because a lot of people go to it. It is an evening meeting, which means it will likely be better attended than morning or afternoon meetings, and people have told me they usually have interesting speakers. It is also a "century meeting," meaning that though it is an open meeting, the speakers and topics will orbit around the experiences of members who either have lost or want to lose at least 100 pounds. It is also a "speaker's meeting"; thus, most of the meeting will be focused on one person's telling of his or her personal story. This meeting, like many, is in a church basement. The room is large with a low ceiling and pillars throughout. Though there are at least fifty people already present, I am surprised at how quiet the room is. People mill about and greet each other, but the mood is calm, almost reverent. In the far corner there is a table with decaffeinated coffee and tea set out along with paper cups and artificial sweetener, but no milk, creamer, or sugar. Next to this table is another table of Overeaters Anonymous literature, free brochures, "newcomer" packets, and books and tapes for sale.

With a cup of tea in hand, I sit down toward the back of the room. Two sections of about thirty folding chairs, separated by an aisle down the middle, are arranged in a semicircle, facing a conference table. At smaller meetings, people often sit around one table facing each other, but the larger meetings usually have an arrangement similar to this one. Promptly at 8:00 P.M. the meeting begins. Marvin, the leader, a thin, white male in his fifties, opens the meeting with the Serenity Prayer and then asks for a volunteer to read the "Invitation to Overeaters Anonymous."[14] The fifth step, which states, "We admitted to God, to ourselves, and to another human being the exact nature of our wrongs," is read, and Marvin reminds us that this is a century meeting and all of the service positions at this meeting are filled by persons who have firsthand experience of morbid obesity.[15]

Tonight's speaker is Kelly, an Overeaters Anonymous member for over six years. Kelly is a white man in his fifties, married, and a successful lawyer. Kelly tells his story, how he used to think that what he had was a "weight problem" but that over the years he realized it was something bigger than that. Kelly eventually went to a therapist to talk about his bingeing, but the therapist was "disgusted" and shamed Kelly. Kelly tried several other therapists until he unintentionally found one who had been a member of Overeaters Anonymous for twenty years. According to Kelly, "this therapist had something I wanted."[16] It took Kelly four years with that therapist to go to his first Overeaters Anonymous meeting, and he was actually inspired to do so after attending a Narcotics Anonymous meeting with a friend. He tells us how much sense that meeting made to him. "It was so simple, if they had a problem they couldn't solve, they would use the twelve steps. If I had a problem, I would eat. It was then that I realized that I had a disease, that I was an addict."

Kelly tells us about his first year in Overeaters Anonymous and his ups and downs and his trouble with the spiritual component of the program. Eventually, he resolved this and now says, "I pray for abstinence because it works, not because I believe in God." Kelly has now had five years of abstinence. He eats three "reasonable" meals a day, no sugar, no snacks, no fast food, no wheat or wheat products, and he says abstinence is "beyond my wildest dreams." Nevertheless, Kelly cautions that he never takes his abstinence for granted because he is an addict and his brain does not work the way normal people's brains do; he will always have to keep "working the program."

A timer rings and Kelly's share is over. There is time for open sharing, though we are reminded that no "cross-talk" or commenting on another person's share is allowed. Before sharing, we are asked to practice the seventh tradition, which states, "We are self supporting through our own contributions."[17] The leader tells us that only Overeaters Anonymous members should contribute and that the suggested donation is two dollars per meeting. Marvin begins the passing of the basket and time for shares starts. Many issues come up in the shares: people share gratitude for abstinence

and struggles with relapse, but, surprisingly, few of the shares have anything to do with food, something I have also noticed at other meetings.
After twenty minutes, the leader tells us it is time for the meeting to end.
We all stand, hold hands, and again say the Serenity Prayer, this time
"for all those who still suffer."

Founded in Los Angeles in 1960 by Rozanne S., Overeaters Anonymous
is a twelve-step group designed to help people recover from the disease of
compulsive overeating. Overeaters Anonymous was consciously modeled
after Alcoholics Anonymous (AA), using the same twelve steps that AA
has been using to help alcoholics find recovery since 1939. Members of
Overeaters Anonymous begin with the premise that compulsive overeating is not simply a result of a lack of willpower or bad habits, but a chronic
and incurable disease. While the disease of compulsive overeating cannot
be cured, sufferers can find sustained recovery through working the twelve
steps and achieving abstinence. In its over fifty-year history, Overeaters
Anonymous has endorsed a variety of food plans; but since the late 1980s it
has refused to endorse any particular plan, instead suggesting that members create their own food plans with the help of their sponsor or doctor.[18]
Overeaters Anonymous is a nonprofit group and its meetings are free,
although the seventh step suggests that those who can should donate two
dollars per meeting. Newcomers are asked not to contribute until they
have decided if they want to become members. This money is used for pay-
ing rent on meeting rooms (most often in churches, community centers,
and sometimes hospitals) and for printing literature. Overeaters Anonymous publications are sold at meetings, and, at larger meetings, members
can also borrow inspirational audiotapes to listen to between meetings. In
2005, over seven thousand Overeaters Anonymous groups meet each week
in fifty-two countries. Overeaters Anonymous, like Alcoholics Anonymous,
has remained almost unchanged since its inception. The meetings, literature, steps, and traditions have not changed since the 1960s.

The Overeaters Anonymous members I observed and interviewed
were largely middle and upper middle class. I interviewed two men and
twelve women, but the makeup of the meetings tended to be more balanced. Over the course of the twenty-two meetings I attended, I estimate
that 30 percent of the members were men. However, in part because the
common tie between Overeaters Anonymous members is the disease of

compulsive overeating, and not necessarily a desire to lose weight, Overeaters Anonymous literature appears to be fairly gender neutral. Nonetheless, many of the issues shared by women in the meetings I observed surrounded parenting, codependence, and marital problems. Overeaters Anonymous meetings were far more racially homogenous than Weight Watchers meetings. Though the meetings all took place in the same diverse urban area, the vast majority of people I saw at meetings were white, as were thirteen out of fourteen of my interviewees.

The central feature of Overeaters Anonymous is the belief that compulsive overeating is a three-pronged disease over which the sufferer has no direct control.[19] Overeaters Anonymous literature states that compulsive overeating is an "emotional, physical, and spiritual illness."[20] Overeaters Anonymous literature further states that compulsive overeaters are "in the clutches of a dangerous illness" that is not curable, and even those who have had many years of recovery can never be comfortable or safe. Janet, an Overeaters Anonymous member for four years, put it this way: "You know, it's so insidious; we talk about this disease being cunning, baffling, and powerful, and I heard somebody sometime add the word *patient.* Cunning, baffling, powerful, and patient, it just waits for the opportunity to jump back up."

Others, like Paul had to adapt their previous understanding of the category "disease" when they entered Overeaters Anonymous: "I had some issues with it in the beginning. I don't know, I mean I don't know the definition of a disease. I had always assumed it was bacterial or viral or congenital. I believe that my compulsive overeating is not something that I can control by myself and I need help for that and if that is the definition of a disease, then that's what I have."

Although interviewees and list-serve members took a more or less literal approach to compulsive overeating as a disease, all agreed that treatment for and recovery from this illness is a largely spiritual process. This spiritual approach is clear in reading the twelve steps.[21] Recovery in Overeaters Anonymous is arrived at by recognizing one's lack of control over the illness and offering it to their "higher power." Indeed, while Overeaters Anonymous recognizes the three-pronged nature of the disease, the steps themselves bolster the idea of spiritual recovery. The twelve steps, as borrowed word-for-word from Alcoholics Anonymous, refer to a higher power as God, both in the singular and the masculine. However, at meetings and in talking to people, I discovered that there is much latitude for people to decide just what or who their higher power is. While many do, in fact, have a monotheistic Christian God as their higher power, for many, their higher power is less clearly defined. Janet told me in an interview:

> They kept talking about God and most of the meetings are in churches, and I'm not a religious person—spiritual, but not religious—and that made me real uncomfortable that I had to go to a church and hear people talk about God. But the thing that they kept saying was "as you define him or her," that the higher power could be nothing more than the energy of all the people in the room at that time. I was able to hear that piece and say that "if I hold onto that piece, I don't have to be Christian; I don't have to have a god that's sitting up in the clouds; I don't have to buy into anybody here's definition of a higher power. I can define my higher power, and as long as I can accept that that's who is in charge, then I'll be OK."

Janet expressed what many of the people I talked to felt, an initial discomfort with the quasi-religious core of the program and an eventual realization that the point is ceding control to something beyond the self, not subscribing to any particular religious doctrine (Lester 1999; Millman 1980).

There is not much discussion of the etiology of fatness in Overeaters Anonymous, but, generally, it is assumed that people are fat because they have the disease of compulsive overeating. It is possible to be a compulsive overeater and not be fat, but for many (though not all) it is not possible to be fat without also being a compulsive overeater. In one of my interviews I asked Janet, a white woman in her mid-forties who had been a member of Overeaters Anonymous for four years, whether or not she thought a woman could weigh two hundred pounds and not be a compulsive overeater. She said, "I just don't see how that could be. I don't see that; my higher power doesn't create bodies to be unhealthy." This quotation reveals a lot about Janet's assumptions about the relationship between weight and health, but it also echoes what I heard from other Overeaters Anonymous members and in Overeaters Anonymous meetings: it is not possible to be fat and not be a compulsive overeater; being heavier than average is unnatural and unhealthy by definition and is the result of a person's "untreated" compulsive overeating.

Overeaters Anonymous literature does not explicitly make the assumption that being fat is necessarily unhealthy, even as compulsive overeating is understood as a disease. Indeed, Overeaters Anonymous literature only speaks about health in very limited and general terms and steers away from medical language. Although many members suggest that one can be healthy and not be exceptionally thin, "obviously" fat people are not likely to also be healthy. Janet's comment also evokes the idea that her higher power wouldn't create unhealthy people, thereby linking the health discourse of the obesity epidemic with the spiritual base of Overeaters Anonymous. This linkage was rarely made within meetings and Overeaters Anonymous literature, but my interviewees did make this link, perhaps in an attempt to reconcile two competing discourses, one of individual disease and one of social epidemic.

Because Overeaters Anonymous is organized around the disease of compulsive overeating rather than framing obesity as a disease, weight plays a secondary role. Weight, as I argued above, is a symptom of compulsive overeating, not an independent problem. For this reason, Overeaters Anonymous and its members are adamant that Overeaters Anonymous is not a diet program and that weight loss is incidental to the treatment of compulsive overeating.

Many of the people I interviewed compared their experience in different weight-loss programs to their membership in Overeaters Anonymous. It is notable that there is debate among Overeaters Anonymous members as to whether diet programs like Weight Watchers can be used as a "tool" along with, but subordinate to, the Overeaters Anonymous program. While many of the Overeaters Anonymous members I spoke with had been Weight Watchers members in the past, none were active members at the time of the interviews. In fact, all of the former Weight Watchers and current Overeaters Anonymous members I interviewed cited their participation in Weight Watchers as part of their denial of the true nature of their eating problems. However, there were a couple of active Overeaters Anonymous and Weight Watchers members who would post to the Overeaters Anonymous list serve I observed. These people would generally refer to the Weight Watchers program as a tool but emphasize that their Overeaters Anonymous–defined abstinence remained primary.

Indeed, it is not uncommon for Overeaters Anonymous members to talk about more conventional diet strategies as tools to help them work the Overeaters Anonymous program. Often people new to the Overeaters Anonymous list serve would mention also being on another weight-loss program and were always warned by others to make sure not to lose the focus of Overeaters Anonymous while employing other means for weight loss. Some Overeaters Anonymous members sought out surgical weight loss. At one meeting I attended, Marcie spoke about her experience in Overeaters Anonymous.[22] As she spoke, she passed around a photo album with her before-and-after pictures and told us about her experience as a compulsive overeater. For Marcie, she was never able to achieve abstinence in her early years in Overeaters Anonymous (she had been a member for five years), so eighteen months earlier she had decided to have gastric-bypass surgery as a tool to help her find abstinence.[23] She said it helped her not only to lose weight, but to achieve the emotional, physical, and spiritual abstinence that eluded her. Given the no cross-talk rule, no one in the group offered any comments on the surgery.

Other Overeaters Anonymous members had weight-loss surgery before joining the group. I never heard one of these people speak at a meeting, and none of my interviewees had had surgery. However, on the list serve, there were often posts by people who had had weight-loss surgery and who nevertheless found themselves in need of help from Overeaters Anonymous. Most of these people had experienced regain some time after their surgery, and this regain helped them realize, as one poster put it, "that the true nature of my disease couldn't be taken care of surgically."

Food: Abstinence versus the Low-Point Binge

Two main themes arise in my data, and both point to clear differences between these two programs that might otherwise be seen in the same category. Both of these programs see themselves as nonmedical in nature, but this behavioral focus manifests itself in two central themes that are at the core of the differences between Overeaters Anonymous and Weight Watchers.

In understanding the experience of members of these groups with weight issues and weight-loss attempts, what is clear is that while there is a common acceptance that to be fat is bad and to be thin is good, the experiences of these people are shaped far more by their particular histories with weight and the philosophies of the programs they participate in than by the sense that obesity is a social problem that they have a moral responsibility to help solve. The underlying philosophies of the two groups reveal themselves through the practices and experiences of Weight Watchers and Overeaters Anonymous in regards to how each group deals with food and how each group understands the etiology and treatment of weight issues.

Though people are allowed to talk about specific foods in Overeaters Anonymous, they often don't.[24] When people do talk about food, it is generally in the course of describing a binge or break in abstinence. At one particularly intense 7:00 A.M. meeting, a very fat African American woman came in after bingeing all night, declaring that she was trying to maintain a two-hour abstinence. Overeaters Anonymous has no set food plan, and people devise their own plans of eating and focus on giving up trigger foods and maintaining abstinence. These plans usually revolve around three meals a day, and many people avoid trigger foods like refined sugar and simple carbohydrates. Overeaters Anonymous food plans often appear to outsiders to be very rigid, but, according to members, they are designed to give people freedom through control, that is, you don't really have to think about food because you no longer have to decide what to eat because your food plan is set.

Janet, an Overeaters Anonymous member, explains how this approach to food differs from that of other diets, specifically Weight Watchers: "[Food] is secondary. It really is, and I think that's the difference between Weight Watchers and Overeaters Anonymous. Weight Watchers is all about, What are you putting in your mouth? How many of those are you going to put in your mouth? Overeaters Anonymous is about, I cannot control this; I gotta let it go and turn it over to somebody else who can, because I can't." This sentiment echoes what Marcia Millman found in her study of Overeaters Anonymous: "One could argue that being fat is the least of the troubles Overeaters Anonymous members face. But for many, being fat comes to symbolize what is wrong in their lives" (1980, 44).

Janet says that, for her, programs like Weight Watchers inspire guilt because they make you feel bad if you look over your journal at the end of the day and discover that you've cheated. She describes her Overeaters Anonymous plan of eating as more proactive and less guilt inducing because she starts the day off planning what she will eat and then sticks to that:

> I loved that all of the diets up until Overeaters Anonymous had me keeping food journals. Like, at the end of the day, write down every-thing you ate. Well, great, I didn't eat what I was supposed to eat and now I'm going to write it down so I can beat myself up even more about what I ate that I shouldn't have eaten. I shouldn't have had those M&Ms, I felt guilty when I picked them up off the shelf, I felt guilty when I bought them, I felt guilty when I ate them, and now I'm going to put them in a journal and feel guilty about it! The first thing my sponsor said to me was "What are you going to eat today? I want you to write down what you are going to eat and tell me what it is." It was a change to "tell me what you're going to eat and then stick to that today; that's what you're having today," not, "Let's look back at your day and beat you up." When I first started, it was like, "Oh, I hate food journals." This is not a food journal; this is "What are you going to have today?" And today, that's what you are going to have.

Ironically, though the idea is to be free from food compulsion, Overeaters Anonymous members constantly think about food, often in the context of determining whether or not they have been "abstinent."

The concept of abstinence in Overeaters Anonymous occupies much the same place for compulsive overeaters as the concept of sobriety does for alcoholics in Alcoholics Anonymous (Millman 1980). Coming up with an exact definition of abstinence is difficult because, as most members of Overeaters Anonymous will tell you, "abstinence is an individual thing." For the most part, however, abstinence is the cessation of compulsive overeating. The closest Overeaters Anonymous as an organization comes to putting forth a specific definition of abstinence is shown in the following excerpt from the "About Overeaters Anonymous" section of the official Overeaters Anonymous website: "The concept of abstinence is the basis of Overeaters Anonymous' program of recovery. By admitting inability to control compulsive overeating in the past and abandoning the idea that all one needs is 'a little willpower,' it becomes possible to abstain from overeating—one day at a time."

Nonetheless, there are patterns in just what abstinence looks like for Overeaters Anonymous members. As a rule, most people include abstaining from their specific "binge" or "trigger foods" in their personal definition of abstinence. Most will say that they abstain from snacking and eating at "problem" times and eat only three meals a day. For most, abstinence includes abstinence from sugar and white flour, and for some this extends to include all forms of wheat and artificial sweeteners.

The degree to which people abstain from these substances varies widely. Most will eat something in which sugar or corn syrup is listed lower than fifth on an ingredient list, while others abstain from all artificial sweeteners, including diet sodas and sugarless gum, as well as honey and other natural sugars. As for wheat abstinence, many members avoid all wheat products, including whole wheat breads and cereals. It is more common for people to simply abstain from processed wheat or white flour. One woman wrote to the e-mail list, concerned about breaking her wheat abstinence by eating a communion host at church. It was pointed out by another list member that, if she is Catholic, given the doctrine of transubstantiation, she does not believe the host is bread, but actually the body of Christ and, therefore, she is still abstinent. If she were to knowingly eat the same communion host before it was consecrated, that might constitute a break in abstinence. Another list member, a leader in another Christian denomination, responded, given his wheat abstention, "I just fixed it so I can't take communion at all! . . . In the future, I'll be able to bless and distribute the gifts [communion] but not partake."

In a similar discussion, Elaine posted the following question to the list: "I have a question about toothpaste. I notice that a little while after I brush my teeth at night I feel hungry and this happens night after night after night. Has anyone else experienced this and is there a certain toothpaste I can buy that won't have this effect on me?" No one else on the list said that they had a specific problem with toothpaste, though many professed to having problems with artificial sweeteners. However, list members responded that if toothpaste did prove to be problematic, she should use baking soda to brush her teeth.

These examples may seem extreme, and they are certainly not representative of what abstinence is for all Overeaters Anonymous members. However, they do illustrate the extent to which the individual definition of abstinence allows members to discipline and regulate the self even in the absence of a rigid program structure. The idea that one could eat problem foods in moderation is seen as a sign of denial because a true compulsive overeater does not have the ability to eat any of their binge foods in moderation. This focus on moderation is very much a part of the "diet mentality" against which Overeaters Anonymous defines itself and its program.

Perhaps more representative of the approach my interviewees took to abstinence is what Janet told me:

> That [the definition of abstinence] is something that Overeaters Anonymous struggles with. People in Overeaters Anonymous struggle with that: "Am I abstinent if I had an extra grape?" I think that comes back to, How are you relating to the food? I could get very obsessed with, you know, one tablespoon of butter and no milk in my coffee. I could really just live for following my food plan, or I could have a food plan and live my life. Some people, in order to be able to live their lives, need to have an enormous amount of structure. In order to be able to live their lives and not think about the food and not be obsessed, they have to know exactly what they're going to eat every meal, every day, to the nanogram. That would be more along the lines of an alcoholic: "Don't drink no matter what; follow this exact food plan no matter what." For me, that degree of control would make me crazy. I don't need that. I am able to find serenity and gratitude and peace within my life and the ability to show up and be present and be pleasant to be around.

So, ironically, for many Overeaters Anonymous members, planning their eating is the key to managing an obsession with food and eating.

Although Overeaters Anonymous very closely follows the structure and philosophy of Alcoholics Anonymous, the comparison of abstinence to sobriety is often difficult because one must consume food in order to survive, thus making abstinence a far more contested category. Some members of both groups feel this often allows people to take the effects of compulsive overeating less seriously than the consequences of alcoholism. Alan, a member of Alcoholics Anonymous for ten years and Overeaters Anonymous for four years, made this observation about the difference between the two groups:

> For me, I think it helps that I'm in Alcoholics Anonymous because you can't just slip in AA [like many do in Overeaters Anonymous] and have the world forgive you. . . . I think AA takes their sobriety, I think, more seriously than people [in Overeaters Anonymous] take abstinence because, ultimately, it is easier to understand the consequences of being drunk; you're going to lose your job and all that. But you know, there are consequences to somebody weighing three hundred pounds. There are lots of consequences; I mean, you're killing yourself. I'm not suggesting that people should be punished for not being abstinent. I certainly wouldn't say that, but I think failure in Overeaters Anonymous is more acceptable to people than it is in AA. I mean, if I just keep "going out" over and over again in Alcoholics Anonymous, people are going to get disgusted, yet in Overeaters Anonymous there's lots of people like that. I don't want people to be punished, and I know that I've been given a gift of abstinence being easier for me, but I don't know, end of sermon, I just wish people in Overeaters Anonymous took the health consequences of being overweight more seriously.

While many see the two programs as similar and use the same language to talk about food and alcohol addiction, there is a tacit understanding among most members that these two addictions differ in ways that make the attainment and maintenance of abstinence very different in either group.

Abstinence, however it is defined, is to many members the single most important thing in their lives (Millman 1980). Without this abstinence they feel incapable of loving themselves or others. An anonymous testimonial printed in an Overeaters Anonymous publication put it this way: "With abstinence a new person emerges. We come to love ourselves and the world around us . . . [and] abstinence is essential for compulsive overeaters. Once broken, even for a short period, the old person we left behind comes back. It is actually an act of love toward ourselves and others, rather than selfishness, to make abstinence the most important thing in our lives without exception" (Overeaters Anonymous 1993).[25] Abstinence, then, brings a whole new person into being with a whole new purpose in life. This contrasts directly with Weight Watchers, where the reason for weight loss is to blend seamlessly in to one's existing life and subjectivity, not to alter it.

One thing is clear; abstinence is not just staying away from certain foods or following a food plan. Abstinence is the "freedom from food obsession" that comes only through working the twelve steps. If members manage to follow their meal plan but are not free from food obsession, then they have not achieved true abstinence, but rather what many refer to as "white-knuckle abstinence." In this type of abstinence, one is not compulsively eating, but the threefold nature (physical, spiritual, emotional) of the disease is not being addressed. One of my interviewees, Jason, a white male in his late thirties and a member of both Alcoholics Anonymous and Overeaters Anonymous, likens this kind of abstinence to being a "dry drunk" in AA. For Jason, a dry drunk is an alcoholic who stops drinking but hasn't really dealt with the reasons why she or he became an alcoholic in the first place. Thus, abstinence, like sobriety in AA, is much more than not eating certain types and amounts of food; it is a state of being in which someone is considered "in recovery" from food obsession and compulsive overeating.

Breaking abstinence is a frequent topic on the list serve, in meetings, and among my interviewees. Most people measure their abstinence in days, though some measure it in years, and many, in minutes and hours. Definitions of what it means to break abstinence are as varied as definitions of abstinence itself. Susan, a forty-five-year-old white woman and member of Overeaters Anonymous off and on for twelve years, defines abstinence as three weighed and measured meals a day and no snacks. Susan also abstains from all forms of sugar, including most fruits, wheat products, including pasta and bread, and rice, potatoes, and peanut butter. After losing over eighty pounds on this food plan, Susan consulted with her sponsor about adding some fruit back into her food plan, and with her sponsor's blessing she added in grapes in a measured portion. Susan had been abstinent for many months by the time she described to me a "slip" that caused her to lose her abstinence: "Then I discovered frozen grapes; they tasted like little bites of sorbet but without the sugar. You have to really watch out for the craving foods. So, I put grapes in the freezer, and then I ate a bunch of them. It was probably about one cup or a little more, which is what I thought it was supposed to be, but the serving size was actually only a half a cup. So, (a) I didn't measure, and (b) I didn't really follow what I thought it was anyway; that was a break in my abstinence."

Others have far less stringent definitions of what constitutes a break in abstinence than Susan. Eating a binge or trigger food is almost always considered a break in abstinence. Eating a slightly larger portion of "clean" or abstinent food may or may not be considered a loss of abstinence, depending on the interpretation of the person and the sponsor.

The Weight Watchers orientation to food implies that it is normal to crave "bad" or "unhealthy" food, that it is normal to actually eat these foods, and that it is normal to want to eat for emotional reasons, especially for women. This orientation reflects a program in which members don't necessarily see either food or emotion as a problem; only the amounts and types of food are at issue. Indeed, given careful planning, one can stay fully within the confines of the Weight Watchers plan and still feel like they are "indulging." With Overeaters Anonymous, on the other hand, food is an addictive substance and must be tightly controlled to avoid relapse into an active disease state. Food is only a "drug of choice" arbitrarily selected from any number of possible addictions (and often existing alongside them).

Food is everywhere at Weight Watchers. Weight Watchers magazines, meeting rooms, and cookbooks are replete with a sort of "food pornography," pictures of modified recipes that look like their more sinful relatives. In meeting rooms, giant pictures of ice cream sundaes made with fat-free frozen yogurt and low-sugar chocolate sauce are next to pictures of one-point salads; and while waiting for meetings to begin, women pore over brightly illustrated recipes in Weight Watchers cookbooks.

Although Weight Watchers officially encourages distributing one's points in such a way that they allow for three meals a day with five servings of fruits and vegetables and at least two servings of low-fat or nonfat dairy products, some members will use all their points at one sitting and eat only zero-point foods (mainly vegetables and non-caloric condiments like mustard and vinegar) for the rest of the day. Jerome tells the story of another man in the meetings he attends at his workplace:

> There's this guy who comes in every week, and he always has this massive vegetable burrito and he says, "OK, this is all I'm going to eat today." And he eats the whole thing during the meeting. He just says he likes to have big meals, so he only eats one per day. He comes in every week, and he'll tell us, "Oh, I went to Costco, and they have these vegetable patties with only so many points and you can eat the whole box." Or he found those "Skinny Cow" ice-cream bars, and he'll just eat a whole package and that's all he'll eat in a day, but he still stays in his point range. I guess I wouldn't want to eat that way.

Most Weight Watchers members I spoke with ate a more varied diet than the man Jerome told me about, but most of them also told me that, like this man, they too search for lower-point-value foods that will satisfy their need to feel like they are eating a big meal or eating something "rich" or "sinful." Members encourage this as well. At one meeting, Deidre was excited to tell us that she had found caramel-flavored mini rice cakes at a local market and that you can eat fourteen of then for only two points; she concluded by saying that the crackers are "just sweet enough to make you think you're eating something good."

This possibility of a "low-point binge" is part of the reason Overeaters Anonymous members don't feel that Weight Watchers as a program addresses the true nature of compulsive eating in the same way their program does. At one of the Overeaters Anonymous meetings I attended, a woman addressed exactly this issue when she said that she had stopped eating her "problem foods" but eventually would find herself bingeing on things like broccoli and celery sticks and needed to incorporate this problem with large volumes of any food into her Overeaters Anonymous food plan. In Weight Watchers, on the other hand, it wouldn't be a problem to eat large quantities of broccoli or celery because they are both zero-point foods that people are encouraged to eat at those times when they want to eat something but aren't really hungry or have already used up their points for the day.

Weight Watchers does encourage members to interrogate their reasons for eating or craving a particular food, not because those reasons are inherently problematic, but because when trying to stick to a daily allotment of points it is a useful exercise. Several of my interviewees used the acronym H.A.L.T. (hungry, angry, lonely, or tired) to describe how they evaluate their feelings when they eat. One of my interviewees, Diane, told me that she thinks of the acronym every time she is about to put something in her mouth: "I ask myself, Am I going to eat this because I'm hungry, or am I angry, lonely, or tired? I may still eat it even if I'm not really all that hungry, but at least I'll know why."

For Weight Watchers it is enough to know why one is eating something and to, if possible, arrange one's points in such a way that a person remains within his or her daily limit. In Overeaters Anonymous, compulsive overeaters lack the control to even accurately evaluate these reasons and so must stick to the food plan "no matter what" to avoid a break in abstinence.

Normative Pathology versus Unique Disease

The two dramatically different perspectives on food and eating at the core of Weight Watchers and Overeaters Anonymous are crystallized in the contrast between abstinence and the low-point binge. Weight Watchers members and the program itself are organized around what I call a model of *normative pathology*. This model assumes that women are more likely to have problems with food and eating than men and that the problem arises when women cannot control this pathological relationship to food in a way that prevents them from gaining weight. That both emotional eating and dieting are simply a part of the everyday experience of being a woman is built into the Weight Watchers program. Weight Watchers does not encourage members to see their food issues as unique or indicative of a disease state, but rather to see them as normal parts of life that can be managed without great upheaval. The solution is to reduce calories, rationalize eating, and be vigilant about monitoring food intake.

Weight Watchers is designed to allow members to appear normal in their eating habits. While individual members may or may not choose to make public their membership in Weight Watchers, the program is organized so that one can theoretically hide the fact that they are dieting or on a new eating plan. They can appear normal in public, cook and eat with their families, yet internally they are counting points, saving points for special occasions, weighing and measuring everything they eat behind the scenes, or writing it down in their journal. Many Weight Watchers products are designed to be discreet, such as pocket point calculators and restaurant guides, pedometers, and bracelets on which you can count your points throughout the day by moving a heart-shaped charm along a string of imitation pearls. Having a problematic relationship to food and weight is plain and simply just part of being a woman, and managing food can similarly be a part of everyday life. This is the case in a social sense, such as having to cook for families and eating out, but also in a more biological sense in that women's desires for food, cravings for particular foods, and emotional eating are simply part of women's natural cycles.

Where this normative pathology becomes problematic is when it "goes too far" and contributes to epidemic obesity. Because the preparing of food and feeding of families is also considered to be part of women's normal relationship to food, women's normative food pathology, alongside a culture of obesity, is central to the spread of obesity. While the racialization of obesity is not as clear in Weight Watchers as it is in the media, Weight Watchers promotes an implicitly white, middle-class style of eating that assumes a nuclear family with access to a wide variety of healthy foods and time to prepare them.

Weight Watchers also promotes itself to women as a way to help make their families and children healthier. Leaders remind us that we aren't just doing something for ourselves, that Weight Watchers recipes are recipes you can "feel good about feeding your family on." Thus, the connections among women, weight, and children are fairly obvious in Weight Watchers. Consider the following interaction at a Weight Watchers meeting. Sherry, the leader, said that a nice offshoot of the program is that it can inspire us to feed our families better. Enid agreed and lamented the poor eating habits of children and how it makes her sad to see families giving their kids sugar sodas and candy. Marianne, a lifetime member, talked about diabetes and how it is an epidemic of a preventable disease. Sherry asked in bewilderment, "Why would you choose to have a disease you can prevent?" Sherry then transitioned back to that day's planned program and told us how to make a three-point treat using frozen biscuit dough and fat-free pudding.

Several of my interviewees said that part of their reason for wanting to lose weight is to "be a good example" to their children about how to relate to food, showing concern about preventing food issues in their children. This concern for being an example to others is not present in Overeaters Anonymous because of the individualized focus of the notion of compulsive overeating as a unique disease. A person's disease negatively impacts others because, without abstinence, one cannot be a good partner, parent, child, worker, or friend because compulsive overeating is controlling his or her life. For a member of Overeaters Anonymous, compulsive overeating as a disease does not have the element of contagion that the pathological eating of a Weight Watchers member might have as he or she passes on certain eating habits to the children.

The majority of Overeaters Anonymous members I talked to said that obesity is a symptom of the disease of compulsive overeating, not a disease in and of itself, thus distancing them from seeing themselves as part of an epidemic yet maintaining their self-identification as addicts suffering from a specific disease. Compulsive overeating is a loosely defined term; some people identify as compulsive overeaters because they have a long history with bingeing, dieting, and food obsession. They say that the disease has cost them their jobs, families, health, and sense of self and has ruined their lives. Most Overeaters Anonymous members agree that some people are compulsive overeaters and some are not; the designation is largely subjective for those who are normal weight or only slightly overweight, although for those who are truly fat, the diagnosis is often assumed.[26] Either way, the disease is an individual psychological malady often indicative of deep flaws; it is not, first and foremost, a social disease of a specific historical moment, thus distancing Overeaters Anonymous from the obesity epidemic.

Conclusion

Given its focus on the normative food pathologies of women and its situating of these within the discourse of a culture of obesity, Weight Watchers members are far more likely to see themselves as part of the obesity epidemic than are Overeaters Anonymous members, who see themselves as uniquely diseased and outside of the social flux of the epidemic. Weight Watchers eschews the language of disease used by Overeaters Anonymous, but its view of obesity is actually more in line with current thinking on obesity, seeing it as the outcome of culture of obesity.

The *normative pathology* model of Weight Watchers assumes that overeating and obesity are a normal part of female existence. Not only are women pathological in and of themselves, but, as mothers and feeders of the family (Boero 2009; DeVault 1991), they are in a unique position to either further or arrest the spread of the epidemic. People are fat because they have learned bad habits and because we live in a culture of obesity in which high-calorie, high-sugar, and high-fat foods are often cheaper and more convenient than healthier foods. Rather than focusing on disparities in access to nutritious foods and health care, programs like Weight Watchers focus on getting women to rationalize the process of eating through counting, measuring, and weighing.

In Overeaters Anonymous, on the other hand, members do not see themselves as part of a social trend toward "dangerous" levels of fatness because they see themselves as uniquely diseased and addicted. This psychological and spiritual flaw is ahistorical; most of the people I interviewed believed they would be compulsive overeaters no matter where or when they were born. This discourse of obesity does not allow for Overeaters Anonymous to so easily absorb the language of the obesity epidemic the way Weight Watchers has; rather, it places the compulsive overeater outside of this particular historical moment.

Though the goal of the compulsive overeater is a normalized body, the unique disease model of Overeaters Anonymous does not seek to normalize people's subjectivity in the same way that the normative pathology model of Weight Watchers does because the abnormality of the compulsive overeater is fixed and unchangeable. Nonetheless, the fixed abnormality of the compulsive overeater in Overeaters Anonymous serves a purpose within a system of disciplinary power; the permanently abnormal are necessary for the large majority of us to be able to identify ourselves as normal or as capable of achieving normalcy.

In the context of the obesity epidemic, this distinction is important because if compulsive overeating is and has always been by and large the same disease, then the compulsive overeater is no more or less a part of the obesity problem than before obesity came to be seen as epidemic. Even with policy makers and medical experts appealing to people's sense of personal and social health to intervene into the epidemic, it is unlikely that Overeaters Anonymous will change its orientation to weight. On the other hand, Weight Watchers bases its understanding of food, weight, and weight loss on a model that, like characterizations of obesity in the media and public health literature, draws on commonsense notions of gender, food, and weight in a way that allows it to be flexible in its adjustments to popular discussions of the obesity problem without fundamentally compromising its core program.

Weight Watchers and Overeaters Anonymous are both long-established and well-known programs whose members' experiences attempting to lose weight occur in the context of an obesity epidemic and reflect both the changing discourse of obesity and the persistent frameworks of the two groups. But what about newer interventions into obesity, treatments like surgical weight loss, designed to be both quick and dramatic ways to quell the rising tide of obesity? In the next chapter, I look to the case of bariatric or weight-loss surgeries. What accounts for the increasing popularity of these surgeries? How do individuals experience the rapid physical and emotional changes that happen as a result of these surgeries, and what happens when these surgeries fail?

4

Bypassing Blame

Bariatric Surgery, Normative Femininity, and the Case of Biomedical Failure

As with the construction of the obesity epidemic and the experience of people in traditional weight-loss programs, notions of normalcy and techniques of normalization are central to the popularity of weight-loss surgery and the experiences of those who have sought out surgical weight loss. Yet the desire of patients to achieve a sense of being *normal* is often curtailed by the physical realities of the post-surgical body as well as normative expectations of gender and sexuality and a more overarching location of the problem of weight within the individual.

To be sure, weight-loss surgery is but one intervention into the obesity epidemic. More traditional behavior modification and fitness programs like those discussed in the previous chapter have been reframed to address the epidemic while maintaining the original focus of each program. In addition, research on and development of new weight-loss drugs, slowed in the mid-1990s by the fen-phen scandals (Mundy 2001), has expanded dramatically in recent years (Campos 2004). Attention to epidemic childhood obesity and calls for public health and legislative interventions into things like school nutrition and soft drink consumption can be heard almost daily. However, weight-loss surgery is unique among these interventions not only because it permanently changes one's anatomy, but also because it is the most dramatic, expensive, and rapidly spreading obesity treatment available.

On the surface, weight-loss surgery may seem to be a cut-and-dry example of the operation of medical authority in which clinicians define a disease (obesity) and treat it surgically. The ability of the medical profession and professional obesity groups like the American Obesity Association (AOA) and the North American Association for the Study of Obesity (NAASO) to classify obesity as a disease to be treated surgically hinges on the interaction of conventional norms of gender, race, health, and sexuality. In turn, the citation of these norms in the case of weight-loss surgery, both pre- and postoperative, is possible because of what we *know* about fat people, namely, the commonsense understandings of the personalities and inner lives of fat women.

Bariatric Surgery

The medicalization of obesity is nowhere more evident than in the popularity and urgency surrounding the development of bariatric or intestinal-bypass surgeries. There are several varieties of weight-loss surgeries, but all in some way involve sealing off or removing most of the stomach to limit food intake or bypassing parts of the intestines to prevent food absorption. In the face of an epidemic, these surgeries, designed to treat the most extreme cases of morbid obesity, are becoming more and more common. The American Society for Metabolic and Bariatric Surgeons (ASMBS) estimates that in 2009 more than 220,000 of these surgeries were performed in the United States alone.[1] This is up from 16,200 in 1992 and 36,700 in 2000 and 140,600 in 2004.[2] The ASMBS estimates that over 80 percent of these surgeries are performed on women.[3]

The most common type of weight-loss surgery is the Roux-en-Y gastric bypass, frequently referred to as a *gastric bypass* or RNY. In the Roux-en-Y procedure, the stomach is reduced to approximately 2 percent of its normal size by creating a small pouch or "new stomach." In addition, between three and four feet of the small intestine are then bypassed, and the new stomach is connected below the bypassed intestine segment, at which point digestion is allowed to begin. This procedure facilitates weight loss in two ways. First, as the new stomach holds only one to two ounces, there is an extreme reduction in the amount of food a person can eat. Second, since a large portion of the small intestine is bypassed, fewer calories and nutrients are able to be absorbed. Therefore, the RNY is both a "restrictive" and "malabsorbtive" procedure.[4] Preoperative patients are warned that this procedure has many potential side effects and complications ranging from blood clots, bleeding, hernias, infections, ulcers, and chronic anemia, to constipation, hair loss, vomiting, and weight gain (Kaiser Permanente 2003). The frequency with which any of these side effects occur is unclear due to lack of data, but the number experiencing more serious complications, while likely significantly larger than in other elective surgeries, is relatively small in relation to the large percentage of patients who experience more common complications like vomiting, hair loss, and fatigue.

Why Surgery?

The popularity of weight-loss surgery can be attributed to three main factors. Among the most significant is the visibility of celebrity weight-loss surgeries, like those of singer Carnie Wilson and TV personality Al Roker. Second, individuals choose surgery to remedy or avoid the purported health risks of obesity. Yet even more potent than the public transformation of celebrity bodies or concern for individual health is the promise of normalcy that comes with surgery. This normalcy, or the ability to move through life without one's weight being a defining feature, is the most often cited reason my interviewees gave for having weight-loss surgery, and it is also a desire appealed to by the doctors selling surgery.

The prevalence of celebrities having weight-loss surgery has grown in the last several years, and those like singer Carnie Wilson, once (and again) an outspoken advocate of size-acceptance,[5] now declare themselves to be advocates for morbidly obese persons seeking a surgical solution. Wilson even had her surgery broadcast live over the Internet to raise awareness about the seriousness of morbid obesity (*Obesity Help* 2004). Not only do these celebrities talk about their surgeries in the mainstream media, but specialty publications on weight-loss surgery often feature interviews and photo essays about them and their surgery experiences. One of my interviewees, Alan, told me that though he had heard of weight-loss surgery, it was watching television personality Al Roker talk about his own experience in a television interview that inspired him to begin to research weight-loss surgery and talk to his doctor about having it. Others, like Kathy, are skeptical of the focus on celebrity surgeries: "I think weight-loss surgery is a great thing, but I also think it is dangerous to glamorize it with the focus on celebrities who have done it. I mean, Carnie Wilson has had tons of plastic surgery and probably has a personal trainer too. Your average weight-loss surgery person has all kinds of flabby skin and doesn't have the money to get it cut off." Others shared Kathy's sentiments, yet most people saw these celebrities as role models who brought weight-loss surgery into the mainstream.

Equally central to the popularization of surgical options for weight loss is the sense of urgency that accompanies the designation of obesity as epidemic. This sense of urgency is conveyed through the media, in the medical field, in public health, and, most significantly for individual patients, in informational materials for the surgeries. An example of this is in a weight-loss surgery brochure from a bariatric clinic in Los Angeles. The headline of the overview story is entitled "Surgery for Severe Obesity: Drastic Treatment for a 21st Century Epidemic." In the story, the surgeon details the conditions thought to be associated with obesity and gives statistics on the economic cost of treating obesity and obesity-related conditions. A brochure for a different weight-loss surgery program states in bold on the first page that "both the medical profession and the general public are recognizing the fact that obesity kills." This sense of urgency is furthered by an enduring American faith in the legitimacy and efficacy of surgical and medical intervention.

The presumed catastrophic impact of obesity on individual health is also cited as a reason for surgery. In one informational seminar, Joy, a middle-aged white woman one year out of gastric-bypass surgery, explained to seminar attendees that, in fact, when she had her surgery, she had none of the obesity-related co-morbidities that many surgery patients have. She had no health problems at all. For Joy, her general good health was a main reason for having the surgery. She said, "It is easier for your body to handle surgery when it is healthier, and at the rate I was going it was just a matter of time before I had high blood pressure, diabetes, and all that good stuff."

Indeed, every surgeon I heard speak at an informational seminar or support group said that people who are healthier at the time of surgery have more success and fewer major complications. Yet, ironically, to qualify to have the surgery covered by insurance, patients must have a certain number of co-morbidities or health problems presumed to be related to their weight. One interviewee told me that she and her doctor "basically made up co-morbidities," reporting that she was "pre-arthritic" and "pre-hypertensive." The interviewee quickly followed this statement by telling me that she was "certain that had I stayed fat I would have had all of those conditions anyway." The idea that healthy fat people will inevitably suffer health problems due to their weight bolsters and is bolstered by conventional scientific wisdom that fatness always equates to ill health. Moreover, surgeons would prefer to do the surgeries on people who, while meeting the BMI threshold for surgery, lack the co-morbidities required for insurance approval. According to one surgeon, this would both be easier for patients and "lower the complication rates" associated with the surgeries.

Although it may seem odd to do major intestinal surgery on healthy fat people, it is the risk assumed to be inherent in obesity that becomes the justification for such surgeries. It is taken for granted by surgeons and patients alike that though obese persons may not have any obesity-related health problems at the time of surgery, it is a virtual certainty that without the surgery they would develop them.

Finally, all weight-loss surgery patients have tried traditional diets based on caloric restriction and exercise,[6] and everyone I spoke with cited these diet failures as a reason they sought out weight-loss surgery. Charmaine told me: "At some point, you have taken enough pills, counted enough calories, and drunk enough nasty shakes that you know that it is not going to work. I mean, I tried everything; in the 1970s I even did a diet where I had to drink the urine of pregnant women. Isn't that disgusting? Eventually, you learn that these things don't work and the people who sell them just want to make a buck. I guess the surgeons do too, but at least surgery works." Like Charmaine, many others I spoke with criticized the profit motives of the diet industry. Many felt that the diet industry was guilty of false advertising, of selling a product it knew would only work temporarily, and many saw surgery as a permanent solution.

For most of the people I talked to, however, a more elusive desire to be normal matched or outweighed all other reasons for having weight-loss surgery. To be sure, people's definitions of what it meant to be normal varied. Leann, for example, simply wanted to take part in daily activities without people staring at her or making comments as she walked down the street. For others, being normal meant being able to shop in the regular women's section of a department store or not worrying about the fit of an airplane seat. Being normal meant not having to deal with the social and physical obstacles fat people deal with on a daily basis.

Selling Surgery, Selling Normalcy

The weight-loss surgery community is built around two central commonalities among its members: the experience of living life as a very fat person and the experience of having had or desiring to have weight-loss surgery. These experiences of stigma and discrimination are at the center of fat people's subjectivity. The common experience of having lived life as a fat person in a fat-phobic society is drawn upon by surgeons and surgery advocates in encouraging people to have weight-loss surgery. Surgeons often cite the social, economic, and medical discrimination experienced by most surgery candidates as one of the most compelling reasons to have surgery. Indeed, my interviewees and people I have spoken with informally at weight-loss surgery seminars and events all cite size discrimination as one of their main reasons for deciding to have the surgery. Kate described it this way: "It's like, all of a sudden you can sit in a movie theater seat again, or not get a seat belt extender on the plane. I think thin people take that stuff for granted, but it is really hard to be in the world like that. It is hard to never fit, to have people assume things about you because you're fat. I would be a liar if I said all that wasn't a big consideration going into this."

All of my interviewees experienced weight-related discrimination for a significant portion of their lives and hoped that surgery and the potential resulting weight loss would alleviate some of this suffering and bring them into the realm of the normal or at least the realm of the unremarkable. For many, it was particularly potent to hear an acknowledgment of this discrimination from a doctor, as many who choose weight-loss surgery have had highly negative interactions with the medical profession in the past. Indeed, a number of people I spoke with cited their weight-loss surgeon as the first doctor they had ever had who did not lecture them on their weight or seem disgusted by their bodies. Maya, a thirty-seven-year-old white woman, told me her bariatric surgeon was "the first doctor in my life who touched my body and didn't seem grossed out." In addition, both surgeons and patients expressed a hope that weight-loss surgery could help them appear normal in society and go about life without constantly running into barriers both literal and figurative.

The social benefits of surgery are emphasized in informational materials. One pamphlet from a bariatric surgeon and member of the ASMBS shows anatomical diagrams of two weight-loss surgery procedures. Under these diagrams is written in large print, "Patients no longer face the social stigma or the many indignities attached to obesity." Literature from weight-loss surgery programs most certainly highlights the potential of surgery to bring a person more into line with a normal BMI, but underlying the focus on health and BMI, and potentially more appealing to stigmatized fat people, is the promise of social normality.

Another common experience shared by weight-loss surgery patients in their presurgery lives (and sometimes postsurgery as well) that helps build community is repeated failure at other weight-loss attempts. The moral discourse of obesity has long blamed fat people for their weight and inability to lose weight, despite well-known statistics on diet failure rates (Bacon 2008; Fraser 1998; Schwartz 1986). In sharp contrast, weight-loss surgeons and others in bariatric surgery programs emphasize that people are not fat because they are lazy, undisciplined, or simply eat too much. Informational literature from surgery programs and information given out at informational seminars often emphasize that surgery is an option precisely because willpower has little or nothing to do with people's weight-loss failures. Surgery is necessary because traditional diets don't work and because a large proportion of individual obesity can be attributed to genetics, not behavior. One speaker at the Obesity Help convention echoed a sentiment I heard at all of the informational seminars I attended when he said, "If all we had to do was eat less and exercise to lose weight, then no one would have weight-loss surgery." Thus, diets fail the vast majority of the time because they assume that obesity is simply an issue of food choices and personal behavior. However, according to weight-loss surgery advocates, this misconception accounts for most diet failure and makes surgical intervention necessary.

The attempt by surgeons to move obesity from the realm of moral failure to the realm of biomedicine represents the co-optation of the language of body size long used by fat activists. Writings on the size acceptance movement (Sobal 1999, 1995) suggest that the core assumption of the movement is that fatness is not a moral issue. Rather, for the size acceptance movement, fatness is a political issue; and social, not individual, change needs to happen in order to end discrimination against fat people (Boero 2010; Goodman 1995; Millman 1980; Poulton 1997; Wann 1998). To be sure, there are key differences between bariatricians and fat activists, mainly in terms of dealing with fat phobia at an individual or social level. However, the shared desire to take the focus off of moral failure on the part of fat people represents a co-optation of a central piece of the fat acceptance message in order to normalize the experience of diet failure and make potential patients more comfortable with a profession and procedures which otherwise might be reminiscent of their all-too-common experience of medical discrimination.

The core difference between the biomedical and political efforts to move away from the doctrine of moral lassitude of fat people is that for the surgeons the answer to the problem is internal and involves the permanent surgical alteration of the body, whereas for the size acceptance community the answer lies in accepting oneself as a fat person, normalizing the existence of differently sized bodies, and working to change a fat phobic society (Boero 2010; Goodman 1995; Thomas and Wilkerson 2005).

This internalized response to discrimination tacitly endorsed by weight-loss surgeons resonates with Sander Gilman's assessment of the depoliticizing effect of the development of aesthetic surgery in the late nineteenth century. For Gilman (2001, 19), "the political 'unhappiness' of class and poverty, which led to the storming of the Bastille, came to be experienced as the 'unhappiness' found within the body. . . . In the former, it was revolutionary change that would cure the body; in the latter, it was the cure of the individual by which unhappiness would be resolved." The obesity epidemic is replete with examples of fat bodies absorbing much of the criticism that might otherwise be leveled at structural inequality (Boero 2010, 2009). Weight-loss surgery may be the clearest example of the individualizing of social unhappiness through modifications made to the body.

One might view the surgery itself as the greatest technique of normalizing bariatric surgery patients, yet it is in the period after surgery that the layered processes of normalization become most evident. Beyond the experience of living in a fat body, the other major commonality of the weight-loss surgery community is the actual experience of having had weight-loss surgery. There is a sense that the unique experience of being a formerly fat person living in a surgically modified body creates both a body of experiential knowledge and somatic needs and characteristics that only those who have undergone the procedure share and presumably can understand. Indeed, the physical challenges brought by weight-loss surgery are unique and many. Postoperative surgery patients must follow very specific rules and regimens in order to avoid serious complications and to ensure that they experience maximum weight loss in the first nine to twelve months after surgery.[7] My interviews and observations show that after their typical one-month postoperative visit with their surgeon, most patients obtain their nutritional and health-care information from each other and from Internet resources. Indeed, the obesity surgery message boards are often filled with questions about how to deal with "dumping," hair loss, nutritional supplementation, and exercise from people who have not yet asked these questions of their surgeons or primary care physicians.[8]

Postoperative patients, or "losers," often serve as "angels," or primary surgery support, for pre-op patients.[9] While surgeons and the weight-loss surgery community alike emphasize that each person will have his or her own unique experience with the surgery, the angel is presumed to have experiential knowledge of the process that only someone who has gone through the surgery can have. This assumption, along with many fat women's desire to avoid interaction with their primary care physician at all costs, also leads people to do most of their presurgery research online through resources like ObesityHelp.com and other weight-loss surgery message boards before they even ask their doctors for a surgery referral.

The relative absence of bariatric surgeons in the postsurgical period is a large part of what makes the weight-loss surgery community so central to people's post-op experience, learning, and support. Throughout the surgery process, patients may only meet with their surgeons a handful of times.[10] One woman I spoke to met her surgeon only once before and once after surgery, as those were the only visits covered by her insurance. She did not seem to have a problem with this because, for her, "the surgeons do the surgery, but only someone else who has gone through surgery can understand what it's like. I go to the doctor for my regular blood work." But for advice, I go to the message boards." This is a pattern among many people I have spoken with; once they are four to six months post-op, they rely largely on their peers for support and medical and nutritional advice related to their surgery.[12]

Though most of this support takes place online or over the phone, ObesityHelp.com members often travel to meet each other individually or at Obesity Help events such as the convention I attended. Although the website has over 250,000 registered members, it is a tight-knit community, and members respond to requests for help and advice rapidly. Susan, a fifty-five-year-old white woman who had RNY surgery in 2003 and has since lost over one hundred pounds, gave me an example. Susan's insurance company wanted her to have surgery at a specialty bariatric clinic over five hundred miles from her home. Susan's surgery resulted in major complications that kept her away from home and in the hospital for over two months. During this time, Susan's daughter-in-law posted a message to a board for that area, and almost instantly Susan was receiving visitors she had never met but who had all had weight-loss surgery and wanted to support her.

The weight-loss surgery community is built around three central commonalities among its members: the experience of living life as a very fat person, the experience of having had or desiring to have weight-loss surgery, and the experience of having to learn how to live in a new, externally more normal body that is at the same time facilitated by a distinctly abnormal intestinal structure. The common experience of having lived life as a fat person in a fat-phobic society is drawn upon by surgeons and surgery advocates in encouraging people to have weight-loss surgery. As discussed above, patients and surgeons often cite the social, economic, and medical discrimination experienced by most surgery candidates as one of the most compelling reasons to have surgery. The other two commonalities of the weight-loss surgery community are the most significant because they are the axes around which post-op patients learn to negotiate their new bodies at a biological level, to be sure, but it is also where they learn to negotiate a world of normative gender and sexual expectations that they had previously been outside of by virtue of their fatness.

Weight-Loss Surgery, Gender, and Heterosexuality

Alone at a round table tucked in a corner of the large ballroom, I watched lavishly dressed people enter and greet each other. A 1980s cover band played classic favorites and people moved to the dance floor in the middle of the room. At the far end of the room from where I was there were vendor tables set up. Unlike the tables set up in the lobby, these were mostly Avon and Mary Kay tables with some jewelry and clothing vendors mixed in. Against another wall was a bar, though most people seemed to be drinking the ice water that was left on each table. It was Halloween, but with the notable exception of a few standards—ghosts, clowns, and a guy in an enormous inflatable fat suit—the costumes were more reminiscent of a cross between a senior prom and a strip club. Some of the women and most of the men were dressed moderately in cocktail dresses and suits, respectively, but a group of women came in wearing very skimpy dresses, French maid costumes, and one particular woman was wearing nothing but fishnet stockings and a thong bodysuit. These women attracted much of the attention of the relatively small number of men at the dance, and, unlike many post-op weight-loss surgery patients, one would never know by looking at them that they had ever been anything other than model thin.

I was still watching people arrive when Lottie and her sister Meg asked if they could sit at my table. We started talking and right off I learned that Lottie, sixty-three, had weight-loss surgery eight months prior and had lost over sixty pounds. Meg, who had not had weight-loss surgery but was "a weight watcher," was here to support her sister and enjoy the convention. Lottie and Meg were, like me, uncostumed and really just wanted to observe all the young folks having a good time. We sat for a while and commented on various costumes and dresses. Lottie and Meg made several disapproving comments about many of the more revealing outfits. In particular, the woman in the fishnet stockings and thong outraged them. They both wondered aloud why any grown woman would wear that in public. The music was loud, so we all did more observing than talking.

The next day at lunch Lottie found me and made a point to come over and tell me that she had a revelation about the woman in the thong. She told me that she had mentioned the outfit to Karen, the organizer of the convention, and that Karen had told her that "a lot of people having the surgery, they never really got to be teenagers and do teenage things because they were fat, and now that they are thin they go back and do some of those things, especially in a safe place to do so, like this convention." Lottie said she thought it made a lot of sense (though she still didn't approve of many of the outfits we saw last night), and she wanted to share it with me. As it turns out, I would hear similar things from nearly all of my interviewees.

Biomedical and cultural understandings of fatness draw from and reproduce many preexisting truisms about fat and fat people. Like the behavioral programs described in the previous chapter, biomedical treatments for obesity also draw from and strengthen entrenched notions of normative femininity and heterosexuality. Gender, heterosexuality, and their reproduction are, implicitly or explicitly, central to both people's individual choice to have weight-loss surgery and the unparalleled growth of weight-loss surgery as a business and intervention into the obesity epidemic. Others (Dull and West 1991; Negrin 2002) have theorized connections between more clearly cosmetic surgeries and the doing of gender and heterosexuality. Here I show that many of these same processes are integral to the way people in the weight-loss surgery community understand their pre- and postsurgical selves even as they maintain that gastric-bypass surgery is a medically necessary intervention and not a form of cosmetic or plastic surgery.

From my interviews I have identified three intersecting processes at the core of the heteronormative nature of weight-loss surgery:[13] relearning heterosexuality, consuming femininity, and becoming visible. These processes are part and parcel of what makes weight-loss surgery such a popular intervention into the obesity epidemic from the perspective of those who have the surgeries. These processes and their ritual enactment also reveal the layering of normative processes involved in the re-creation of the individual subjectivities and bodies of weight-loss surgery patients.

Rituals of Gender, Rituals of Heterosexuality

Many of my interviewees told me that after weight-loss surgery they had to relearn many taken-for-granted aspects of normative heterosexuality, such as flirting, dating, and having sex. Fat women have been relegated to the world of the asexual and unfeminine and have been seen as seeking to escape heterosexuality or hide their sexuality behind their fat (Millman 1980). This characterization of fat women as asexual certainly resonates with many psychological and popular representations of fat women's sexuality, yet others (Braziel 2001; Klein 1998; LeBesco 2004) have also pointed to the perceived hypersexuality of fat women. Jana Braziel (2001) notes that the association of corpulence with excess and desire has also resulted in images of desperate and insatiably sexual fat women. The existence of these two seemingly opposed images nevertheless reveals that in the modern West, the sexuality of fat women has never been located within the realm of the normatively heterosexual.

Characterizations of fat women's sexuality as deviant resonated with my interviewees. Though many of them had successful romantic and sexual relationships as fat people, almost all cited this as an area of intense readjustment after their weight loss. Leena, a thirty-eight-year-old white woman who lost over 150 pounds in eighteen months, described her experience of getting male attention after losing weight:

> When you're the weight that you were, you have no social life. You may have friends, but you don't have guys looking at you, nothing like that, and then suddenly they are, and you don't know what to do. I have guys chasing me down the street in cars sometimes. I've had that happen three times on Main Street, guys pulling up saying, "Where you goin' baby?" "What's your number?" I'm like, "Huh? Me? Who are you talking to?" You don't know how to handle it. You know, women who have been thin all their lives, they know how to handle it.

Leena at once seemed both distressed at being subject to catcalls from men and also acutely aware and pleased that being the object of this harassment made her a part of that vast array of normal women for whom such experiences are just a part of being female.

The experience of being objectified as a fat woman may be familiar, but the sexual objectification that may come with losing weight was a very new experience for my interviewees. Leena went on to describe her own new social life: "We love to put on our party clothes and flaunt in front of other guys, even when our husbands or boyfriends are around; that's what girls like to do." There are three interesting assumptions present in Leena's statements. First, a social life only counts as such when it manifests as a heterosexual relationship. Second, though Leena herself had been married and had been in other romantic relationships, these did not qualify as authentic relationships if they took place before she was thin. The presumed dysfunctionality of fat women's relationships squares with popular expectations of fat women's sexuality and also suggests that fat women's sexual lives gain authenticity only when their bodies shrink. Third, when Leena expressed that now she could do "what girls like to do," she implied that one of the benefits of weight-loss surgery is being able to partake in normal heterosexual activity, activity that, if one took part in while still fat, would be evidence of desperation or a lack of discretion associated with hypersexual fat women (Braziel 2001).

Another of my interviewees, a middle-aged African American woman, explicitly expressed disgust at the idea of young, fat, African American women's sexuality: "I think of these girls, you know, that have all these rolls of fat and have their titties all hanging out with dresses up to here and all this fat in the back of their leg and thinking that's somehow attractive. It's not, and they just look like they'll go with anyone. It is like wearing your mental health status on your sleeve." This woman's analysis of an image of fat women as hypersexual also evokes a racialized view of fat black women's sexuality that resonates with controlling images of black women as hypersexual, animalistic "Jezebels" (Hill Collins 1990; Hobson 2003; hooks 2003). However, it was not the sexuality of all African American women that was at issue with my interviewee; rather, she was concerned with the "mental health status" of those fat black women who were overtly sexual and unapologetic about it. Thus, images of racialized sexuality interact with the notions of fat women's sexuality not only to frame that sexuality as deviant, but also to indicate mental illness.

Several of my interviewees expressed that it is almost impossible for the heterosexual relationships of fat women to be normal and healthy because there is a de facto pathology on the part of men who are attracted to fat women. Three of the women I interviewed said they felt men dated them when they were fat because they could "control" them or because they felt there would be less competition from other men and less likelihood of the women leaving them. Leena went on to tell me that she thinks that weight-loss surgery often has the secondary effect of helping women get out of bad marriages and relationships because they no longer feel like "they have to settle for some guy who will be with them when they're fat." Leena also said, and I observed, that many couples in which both partners are fat would have weight-loss surgery at or close to the same time. Leena suggested part of the reason couples will do this is so that one person doesn't get jealous of the other when she or he "gets thin."

The high divorce rate after weight-loss surgery is a frequent topic on the ObesityHelp.com message boards. One post proclaims that "after weight-loss surgery you're actually more likely to get a divorce than get a boyfriend!" There is no data on the divorce rate among weight-loss surgery post-ops, yet there seemed to be a consensus on the message boards as well as among my interviewees that fat women stay in bad relationships because of low self-esteem related to their unattractiveness and that, once thin, they have more relationship options open to them and are more likely to leave relationships they no longer feel dependant on. One interviewee explained: "A lot of people go through marital problems when they have weight-loss surgery because, you know, their husbands married a fat lady and they've always known a fat lady and all of a sudden the women become attractive and they are flirting where they've never flirted, and it is threatening."

Thus, the experience of male attention after weight-loss surgery is an adjustment for female post-ops because either they have never had any sexual or romantic interest from men or that attention has been more indicative of a form of male psychopathology and the low self-esteem of fat women than any genuine attraction. Post-op dating, then, is a large part of the normalcy that is the goal of many who decide to have weight-loss surgery.

The weight-loss surgery community does much to help people learn or relearn normative heterosexuality. On the ObesityHelp.com website there are message boards dealing with dating, sexuality, divorce, and even a singles forum where weight-loss surgery patients can meet other single pre- and post-op weight-loss surgery patients. At the Obesity Help convention there are dances and social events like the ball described above. There are areas of the convention like the "new you room," in which women can get tips on fashion and makeup as well as shop for new clothing and get glamour photos taken. There are also more explicit enactments of normative heterosexuality. These ritual enactments within the weight-loss surgery community, such as fashion shows, makeovers, and dances, are often similar in form and function to more generalized heterosexual rituals like weddings and proms. These rituals seek to reinforce the normalcy, invisibility, and rightness of heterosexuality, but they are also important ways for post-op surgery patients to learn how to participate in the normatively heterosexual world as appropriately gendered bodies. The primacy of these rituals is another vantage point from which to see that self-correcting to conventional norms of sex and gender is vastly more significant than norms of health in driving the weight-loss surgery community and industry.

The "post-op fashion shows" at Obesity Help conventions crystallize this ritual enactment. The fashion show happens on the last day of the convention and features models who have all had weight-loss surgery and lost large amounts of weight. The stage at the center of the hotel ballroom serves as a runway, and behind it is a large screen. As the models cross the stage, "before" pictures flash on the screen along with their name, date of surgery, starting weight, and current weight. The fashion show is organized into categories, "career wear," "lounge wear," "active wear," "sportswear," and "formal wear." In each category a man and a woman come out and model as an emcee announces their names and encourages the audience to cheer by asking questions like "Isn't she sexy?" or "Ladies, I have it on good authority he's single."

The outfits modeled in each category reproduce understandings of normative femininity and masculinity as embodied by those of normal size. In many ways the outfits and postures of the models represent fantasies of what being normal would be like. In the career-wear category, Jason, who lost over 200 pounds in nineteen months, modeled a firefighter's uniform (he is not actually a firefighter) to the hoots and hollers of the mostly female audience. As he walked the catwalk in his very masculine boots, jacket, and helmet while holding a hose, the picture of him that flashed on the screen behind the stage reminded us that less than two years ago he weighed well over 400 pounds and spent most of his days on the couch wearing sweatpants. Hardly the heroic, trim, and masculine firefighter we now saw before us. Jason's female counterpart in the category was Maggie, who came on stage wearing nurse's scrubs, and we saw her picture 127 pounds earlier in similar scrubs as the audience cheered. The most notable category was lounge wear. Here we saw Jeb, who, having lost over 350 pounds, was one of the biggest losers at the convention, strut out in a Hugh Hefner–like smoking jacket and silk pajamas. Hanging on his arm was Marley, wearing a much more revealing negligee. Having lost *only* 90 pounds, Marley seemed to have far less of the excess skin that can plague those who lose larger amounts of weight. Striptease music boomed and the audience was on its feet cheering. Jeb pulled open the sash of his smoking jacket and produced a cigar and pretended to smoke it while Marley hung off his arm as they sauntered suggestively off stage, and the fashion show came to a close with thunderous applause.

The fashion show is but one example of how many post-op weight-loss surgery patients are reintroduced to the roles and expectations of normative heterosexuality after having lived on the constitutive outside of acceptable sexuality during their lives as fat people. For the men, being able to model the attire of men who do physically demanding work and come home to scantily clad wives allows them to symbolically enter or reenter their natural place in the social order. For women, the message is that now that they are thinner, they can appropriately test their understandings of normative femininity and sexuality in a space where their sexuality is not ridiculed.

These exaggerated rituals can be likened to the *doing* of gender and heterosexuality in those groups for whom the enactment of gender must be more conscious. Not unlike transsexuals learning the appropriate doing of gender as adults (Schrock, Reid, and Boyd 2005; West and Zimmerman 1987), fat people, particularly women, have often been excluded from normative patterns of gendered behavior, interaction, and embodiment.

Consuming Femininity

"The clothes are the best thing, definitely." This quote is from Arianna, a thirty-year-old Latina who had weight-loss surgery eight months prior to our interview. Having lost 110 pounds in that time, she expressed a sentiment that all nine of my female interviewees shared. For fat women, shopping for clothes can literally feel like negotiating a minefield. The women

I interviewed all shared their angst about finding clothes that fit and all shared their joy at being able to wear normal clothing sizes,[14] and several cited clothes shopping as one of their favorite activities post weight loss. For these women, it was not only about fitting into clothes they previously could not fit into, but also explicitly about feeling able to participate in a stereotypically female activity as a normal female. While Leena's earlier statement was about flirting being "what girls do," Maggie expressed her delight at being able to shop and be "just one of the girls." As she put it, "I used to watch everyone else shop and maybe buy a pair of earrings or something. Now I can actually participate and shopping has become fun."

The new bodily forms created through weight-loss surgery also create new markets for everything from new forms of plastic surgeries to remove post-weight-loss "redundant skin,"[15] to nutritional supplements and specialty foods, to beaded medic-alert bracelets and preorganized weight-loss surgery scrapbooks in which one can chronicle one's weight-loss journey. In and of themselves, many of these products have little or nothing to do with weight-loss surgery, and most of the products are marketed explicitly for women. The example below shows that this new ability to fit into normal female consumptive patterns is promoted by organizations like Obesity Help and is also intimately tied to reproducing an understanding of appropriate gender norms.

On the first morning of the convention we were all again in the ballroom and listening to Jeb, an Obesity Help staff member and weight-loss surgery patient, detail the events of the day. He pointed over to the corner of the ballroom where the makeup and clothing vendors were set up. He told us that in this area, the "new you room," there were clothes, pictures, makeup, jewelry, in short, "a woman's dream." He joked to the women in the room, "You all told your husbands you were going to a conference and now you get to buy stuff!" Everyone laughed. He went on, "Well, guys, there is some men's stuff, but we'll go drink coffee and let them shop." At the same time, Jeb is reinforcing a script in which women go shopping and spend men's money. Shopping is a feminine space a normal man would only enter grudgingly. Getting a cup of coffee and hanging out with other men is "what guys do."[16]

In spite of an inverse relationship between income and average weight (Rothblum 1999), fat people are often seen as poster children for

American overconsumption. Weight-loss surgeons and others are quick to draw on this image in their attempts get people to shift their consumption patterns. At one support group a surgeon suggested that patients learn to "shift your reward systems from food to things you really want." In response, one patient said that she now rewards herself for various weight-loss goals with items of clothing, stating, "My size changes so often now, I almost have to!" While normative femininity may involve overconsumption, for fat women this overconsumption must be expressed more appropriately—through retail.

Becoming Human

For my informants these first two processes culminated in nothing short of what one woman called "becoming human." Knowledge on the part of fat people that they are the outside around which normality is defined has made them feel less than human, literally nonexistent as a subject but rather framed as an object, a cautionary tale, a freak. The ability to participate in society as an average person is one of the most transformative aspects of weight-loss surgery, especially for women.[17] As shown above, heterosexual attention is central to this recognition and visibility, as part of the knowledge of and ability to act in acceptably feminine ways.[18] My interviewees also indicated that it is a more general recognition of one's attractiveness that really makes surgery "worth it." Charmaine described an incident at her boyfriend's office Christmas party:

> We went to this party and I hear him telling me how pretty I am and I'm like "Whatever," and my friends tell me I'm pretty too. But somebody that I don't know that's not an adult, I hadn't had that happen. I was walking across the room, and they had a boutique set up. I went over and I was looking at some gift baskets. I was wearing a long black skirt and a pink sweater. On the bottom of my skirt I felt a tug, and it was the cutest, prettiest, little four- or five-year-old girl. I look at her and I said, "Hi," and she looked up at me and said, "You are so beautiful." I just totally lost it right there. Not because she said I was pretty, but because she didn't know me; she didn't have any reason to say it. She had nothing but her childhood innocence, and for that

little girl to say that to me was the turning point from the day I had my surgery. That was the day I realized this was a good thing I did.

Charmaine described a visibility wholly different from either the compulsory and objectifying visibility or complete invisibility experienced by fat people. The visibility Charmaine describes is one in which she is seen as a normal woman, one who feels respected, and through which weight-loss surgery patients begin to feel they are subjects rather than objects. This visibility and feeling of being fully human, not feeling or being healthier or at less risk of disease and disability, is what made Charmaine happy that she chose surgery. Susan said that one of the most striking things she had noticed post-op was that people would actually look her in the eye. She explained, "It wasn't that strangers said rude things to me when I was fat; they just didn't say anything. They would look and then just look away like they got caught doing something bad or something." She went on to say, "People smile at me now and that feels really good."

The Obesity Help community encourages this feeling of positive visibility. A convention organizer encouraged attendees to have a new professional photograph taken by one of the photographers at the convention by suggesting, "Isn't it time for a new picture? Didn't you always avoid having your picture taken before?" Willingness to have one's picture taken is a huge change for many post-op patients. All of my interviewees talked about not liking to see pictures of them when they were fatter. Many said that literally years of their lives are absent from family photo albums and that they avoid looking at those pictures that do exist except to show them to others as their "before" pictures. The desire to be photographed after surgery shows that it is not only recognition as being human from others, but one's own sense of humanity that changes so dramatically with weight loss.

If the successful surgery patient is one who loses a large amount of weight, keeps it off, follows a strict diet and fitness regimen, consumes clothes but not food, and reintegrates into normal society, then what about those who aren't so successful?

Biomedical Success or Individual Failure?

The official definition of weight-loss surgery success as set forth by the American Society of Bariatric Surgeons defines success as a patient losing and maintaining a loss of 50 percent of their excess body weight over five years. Thus, according to the body mass index (BMI) definitions of over-weight and obese, a person who had surgery at a height of 5 foot 7 inches and 350 pounds would be considered a weight-loss surgery success if she or he lost and maintained a loss of 100 pounds over a five-year period, even though she or he would remain classified as severely obese and still within the BMI range of those eligible for surgery. However, it appears that weight-loss surgery patients themselves would not tend to think of the above example as a success because, at 250 pounds, they would hardly have achieved the normalcy they had hoped the surgery would give them. On a message board for failed weight-loss surgery, one woman who weighed 460 pounds before her RNY surgery and had lost *only* 130 pounds sixteen months postsurgery wrote of just such a situation: "I did not have surgery to weigh 330 pounds. It bothers me a lot to know that my goal weight will still qualify me for WLS. But I have no idea if I will ever even get close to that. Sure, I am glad that I have lost 130 pounds. But in sixteen months that is not what I expected. I do my exercise; I enjoy it. I never expected to be able to weigh 120 like that stupid chart says I should. But I at least wanted something closer to a normal weight than I am now."

This frustration is understandable given the fact that most advertise-ments for weight-loss surgery show patients who have clearly lost signifi-cantly more than 50 percent of their excess weight and in many cases appear to have already gone through plastic surgery to remove excess skin. It is often these people who are invited by their surgeons to speak at weight-loss surgery seminars. Typically, at least one post-op patient from the surgery program being promoted is asked to share his or her story with seminar attendees. The speakers selected by program doctors are usually those who have achieved the most dramatic results, not those who have had the most typical results.

Lenny, the speaker at a public informational seminar to promote a new bariatric clinic at a large suburban hospital, was a forty-five-year-old single white male who, at the time of the seminar, was eighteen months post-op from an RNY procedure. Dressed in form-fitting black jeans and a tight black T-shirt, Lenny looked like the type of guy who had been going to the gym his whole life. In fact, eighteen months earlier Lenny had weighed close to 400 pounds and had never regularly exercised in his life.

Now, at 180 pounds, Lenny worked out at a gym at least two hours every day and often worked overtime at his very physically demanding job as a warehouse worker. He told us he wears compression garments while he works out to help minimize the sagging skin that frequently develops in those who lose weight so rapidly.[19] He was proud to say that he has not had and does not plan to have any plastic surgery to remove excess skin. When Lenny was asked what he eats in a typical day, he told us that for breakfast he eats two scrambled egg whites and water. For lunch he eats a half-cup of white rice with vegetables and soy sauce, and for dinner he eats half a skinless chicken breast and more steamed vegetables. To make sure he is getting his protein in, he also drinks a special protein drink at some point during the day. He told us that he expects that this will be his daily menu for the rest of his life and that he doesn't mind because he feels better than ever and the surgery has saved him from the certain early death he was facing due to his morbid obesity.

Everyone attending the seminar seemed highly impressed with Lenny, and the doctors talked about how proud they were of him and his dedication. One of the surgeons called him "a poster child for weight-loss surgery." A thin man sitting toward the back of the room with his wife (who is considering surgery) asked the doctor if Lenny was representative of most post-op weight-loss surgery patients. The doctor said, "No." She explained that most people do not lose as large a percentage of their weight as Lenny did, and most people will need to have surgical skin removal at some point after their weight loss slows. She said that they chose Lenny to speak because he was an example of "the best of what is possible through weight-loss surgery."

Surgeons will often give potential patients the clinical definition of weight-loss surgery success described above, yet the visual images of success are usually people who have lost a far higher percentage of their starting weight than the average person can expect to lose. It is also the case that post-op speakers at support groups and information sessions and featured in *Obesity Help* magazine tend to be between nine- to thirty-six-months post-op, the period in which most people's weight loss peaks.[20]

There is no more agreement on what constitutes failed weight-loss surgery than there is on weight-loss surgery success. The central medical rationale for having weight-loss surgery is to cure, manage, or prevent conditions such as adult-onset diabetes, sleep apnea, and hypertension (to name but a few), which are assumed to be caused by obesity. However, among weight-loss surgery patients, an assessment of surgical success or failure does not seem to rest on the prevention, alleviation, or abatement of these co-morbidities. For most of the people I talked to and whose stories I read about on the weight-loss surgery message boards, like the woman I quoted above, the success of the surgery seems to rest on having lost enough weight to be able to consider oneself normal.

Most of the online weight-loss surgery chat rooms, list serves, and message boards tend to deal with more of the positive aspects of weight-loss surgery, especially those message boards on the ObesityHelp.com website. Yet there are spaces for people to tell stories of complications, weight-loss surgery failure, and weight-loss surgery regrets. On the Obesity Help.com website there are two such forums, the "weight-loss surgery regrets" message board, and the "2nd time around/weight-loss surgery failure" message board.[21] Most of the people who use these two boards are people who have already had surgery. Occasionally, someone considering having the surgery will post, asking for information about the "downside of surgeries." Most of the people who participate in these two lists seem to know that they are outsiders even in the weight-loss surgery community, both because their surgeries, for whatever reason, were not successful and because they are willing to voice their disillusionment with the surgery. One woman who felt that her surgeon misrepresented the extreme diet and exercise modifications she would have to make after surgery posted the following: "You know, I don't even go to my support groups anymore because I found myself being ignored. . . . I found that I am too blunt, too controversial, and, the truth be told, [neither] doctors nor their staff want people like me speaking up at those groups. I understand why. It's a business, and if I start telling it like it is, from my perspective, from my shoes, it deters people." Few of the people I interviewed or spoke with at the Obesity Help convention brought up the profitability of weight-loss surgery. However, among those who did, all were, like the above poster, people who felt their surgeries had failed or who regretted having had the surgery.

Many on these lists expressed their sense of alienation when attending support groups. Many said that the support groups are basically "preaching to the choir," and some expressed concern for people who feel that if they have had any problems as a result of the surgery, they cannot speak up. One woman gave her impression of the support groups: "Everyone seems all smiles and success stories. I'm happy for them, but I also know somebody in those rooms is having a hard time and is afraid to express any regret about having this surgery." There are perhaps many reasons why criticism of weight-loss surgery is so discouraged by the weight-loss surgery community. Clearly, as the above quotation states, bariatric surgery is, first, a business, and hearing negative experiences may steer potential patients away. Second, many of my interviewees and people I met at events feel defensive about the surgery, believing it is negatively portrayed in the media and that they must correct that negative image through their own positive statements. Third, regret may consciously or unconsciously feel like a futile emotion in those who have had an irreversible elective surgery. This is important because, as I show below, this avoidance of criticism is inextricably connected to how people understand and explain surgical failure.[22] It's also evidence of the enduring quality of the *internalized panopticism* women use to evaluate their bodies and behaviors and through which they develop their sense of self as a project to be worked on (Spitzack 1990).

In the absence of clear surgical error, weight-loss surgery failure, most often defined as the failure to lose at least 50 percent of one's excess body weight or weight regain after surgery, is explained as a result of patient noncompliance, specifically, patients beginning to eat more two years after surgery and, subsequently, "stretching their pouches." This pouch stretching results in an ability to take in more food in one sitting and thus gain weight.

For example, in one breakout session at the Obesity Help convention, a surgeon told the audience that most often weight regain in weight-loss surgery patients is due to patients not continuing to follow the post-op rules of eating once they are past their peak weight-loss stage. According to the surgeon, the rules of eating that must be maintained for successful long-term weight-loss surgery results are as follows: "Eat no more than one bite of food every ten minutes." "Use a stopwatch when eating." And "do not drink liquid half an hour before a meal, with a meal, or for one hour after finishing a meal. Drink no more than one ounce of liquid every five minutes."[23] The surgeon told us that most of the patients he knew who failed did so because they ate or drank too fast. He told us, "There are no scientific studies on this, but if you talk to patients, and they are really being honest, they will tell you that they will eat a half a sandwich in fifteen minutes. . . . We [surgeons] give you this tool, but you have to ask yourself, 'How do I use the tool given to me?' This surgery takes a lot of discipline and learning."

Another surgeon speaking at the convention warned, "If you drink a lot of shakes and high-calorie liquids, then we don't have a surgery for you." A bariatric nurse speaking on the subject of long-term pouch care told us, "Now you have a tool that if you treat it right will last for life. The problem when it doesn't work is that you have the same bad habits that you did before you got it."

Beyond being extraordinarily stringent behavioral prescriptions, these rules are reminiscent of the sorts of regimentation of time, space, and bodies that Foucault (1994, 1977) sees as characteristic of the development of disciplinary power in schools, hospitals, and the military. This regimentation resonates with people's previous experience of traditional dieting, yet at the same time it is assumed by surgeons that in the past people have failed in their internalization of these techniques.

What the above quotations also show is that despite the fact that weight-loss surgeons frequently tell patients before surgery that dieting doesn't work and that their weight isn't their fault, later on in the surgical trajectory, behaviors associated with traditional dieting become the dividing line between those who have long-term weight-loss maintenance and those who regain.[24] These quotes also show that, like the dieter who claims to not be overeating yet still gains weight, weight-loss surgery patients who claim to be following their post-op regimen yet gain or do not lose weight are seen as less than honest with themselves and with their doctors. On the "failed weight-loss surgery" message board, two women expressed their frustration at this assumption. "I am concerned because now I can eat a whole single hamburger with a bun in one sitting.[25] When I told my doctor this, he just said, 'Well, just because you can do it doesn't mean you should.' Please save me from skinny doctors!" In a separate thread on the same message board another woman said: "I was 248 pounds when I had this surgery in late 2003. Eight months later I weigh 174. It has been a full-time job trying to get this weight off, and now I have almost given up.

My doctor says I am 'out eating' the surgery, but I know I am not. No one seems to want to talk to you when you are a WLS failure. They only want to hear the good things." These quotations show that while the success of weight-loss surgery is attributed to surgical skill, patient compliance, and biomedical innovation, failure is seen by doctors as the inability or unwillingness of individual patients to change their behaviors to facilitate weight loss. The assumed lack of motivation or willpower associated with fat people that doctors explicitly criticize in pre-op weight-loss surgery seminars later becomes the comfortably familiar way in which to explain weight gain or failure to lose in *noncompliant* post-op patients.

The specter of the emotional eater also looms large in attempts to explain weight-loss surgery failure. The emotional cater, almost invariably presumed to be female (DeVault 1991; Orbach 1978; Zimberg 1993), is a figure often invoked to explain weight-loss surgery failure. In support groups and at the Obesity Help convention, emotional eating was talked about as one of the most common ways to "eat your way around the tool of surgery." At one postoperative support group I attended, the discussion turned to weight regain and how to avoid it. The surgeon leading the group said that "surgery can take away the calories, but it can't take away the drive to overeat." He said that this was a problem he saw most often in his female patients: "My male patients do better with the surgery than women do. I think this is because they [women] are emotional eaters and men are not. Men eat because they like to eat. I can fix that, but I can't fix emotional eaters."

Many postoperative patients seem to agree with this sentiment. One woman speaking at the convention told the audience that although she regained weight several years after surgery, "my surgery didn't fail me, I failed my surgery." This is perhaps the single most telling statement I heard throughout my research. In suggesting that she could "fail" a surgical procedure, this woman gets to the heart of the individualizing and normative nature of disciplinary power. She went on to explain that though she could never eat much in one sitting, she tried to deal with her emotions by "grazing" and thereby gained back the weight that the surgery had helped her lose.[26] This again highlights that it is patients, not surgeons, who are held responsible for the success or failure of weight-loss surgery and that the *emotional woman* is the cultural trope most easily identified as problematic.

Though surgeons and weight-loss surgery advocates cite well-known statistics on the high failure rates of traditional diets as a justification for weight-loss surgery, when patients are two or more years post-op and their bodies have adjusted to the caloric restriction inherent in most weight-loss surgeries, it is exactly such traditional dieting that is required to maintain weight lost through surgery.

Many of the people I spoke to have done just this. In one support group, Marlene, a middle-aged white woman who had RNY surgery in 2003, told the group that she had started going to Weight Watchers "for emotional support." Marlene had lost 105 pounds in sixteen months, but she knew, "The hard part is still ahead of me." And going to Weight Watchers meetings could help her maintain her weight once she reached her goal. At the time, she could not actively participate in the program as she was unable to eat even close to the minimum number of calories required by Weight Watchers, but she did "listen to people and get tips for later."

Still others have returned to pharmaceutical methods in order to maintain or supplement their weight loss. In response to a message board question about how to keep off weight lost as a result of surgery, one woman who had RNY surgery eighteen months prior told of her own method: "I am taking prescription diet pills to curb my hunger and I haven't gained any weight but I haven't lost any either in six months. . . . I have lost 120 pounds and not a pound more. I do exercise, drink water, and get in ninety grams of protein a day. I also watch my calories and keep them below 1200 a day. I feel like I never even had the surgery and I am just back to dieting again."

The return to dieting after surgery is particularly demoralizing for weight-loss surgery patients who are told by surgeons that dieting doesn't work and who have long histories of failure with mainstream dieting. Others shared techniques like over-the-counter diet pills, liquid diets, and fasting. Still others developed anorexia or bulimia in an effort to stay thin after surgery. In a session on eating disorders at the Obesity Help convention, the leader, a therapist who works with pre- and post-op weight-loss surgery patients, asked the audience, "How many of you have eaten something you knew would make you throw up just to avoid gaining weight?" Several hands went up and the therapist said, "While it is good to be scared of weight gain, being obsessed with it is unhealthy." However, for many, it is unclear where the line between *healthy fear* and *unhealthy obsession* lies.

Even de facto weight-loss surgery spokesperson Carnie Wilson returned to dieting and became the spokesperson for Optifast, a diet program that relies on vitamin supplements and severe food restriction. Wilson got pregnant three years after her RNY procedure and gained a significant amount of weight before, during, and after her pregnancy. Wilson blames her own lack of vigilance for her weight gain. In her online Optifast diary, Wilson wrote, "After feeling disgusted with myself for long enough, I cleaned up my act."[27] Like the woman above who "failed her surgery," Carnie Wilson did not see her weight gain as a reason to question a procedure; rather, she saw it as an individual failure that required a return to traditional dieting to remedy. After regaining the weight lost through Optifast, Wilson appeared on the popular reality show *Celebrity Fit Club*. After continuing to regain weight lost through her extensive efforts, Wilson recently declared in an interview, "You know, after all these years, it's just like we are who we are and it's a struggle for me and sometimes I'm heavier and sometimes I'm thinner" (Shuter 2010).

These reversions to traditional dieting and to individualized moral understandings of success and failure that accompany it are in direct contrast to the biomedicalized, *value-neutral* perspective on weight and weight loss that patients hear from surgeons and others before surgery. However, what this research shows is that earlier and arguably more familiar discourses, even premedicalization discourses of weight and moral failure, are accessible and able to be drawn upon to explain the failure of specialized biomedical interventions. In many ways, the extensive behavioral changes required of weight-loss surgery patients and the many physical side effects of the surgery beg the question of whether gastric bypass is more akin to a surgically enforced eating disorder than it is to a surgical cure for obesity.

Conclusion

Weight-loss surgery as an extreme intervention into the contemporary American obesity epidemic brings into high relief relationships among processes of medicalization, conventional norms of gender and sexuality, and moral discourses regarding bodies and body size. In this chapter I have explored these relationships in three ways. First, I have shown how the popularity of weight-loss surgery relies on the interaction of norms of health, celebrity endorsements, size discrimination, and a general desire to be normal, alongside the sense of urgency surrounding the epidemic. Second, I have looked to the development and rituals of the weight-loss surgery community to show how conventional norms of gender and sexuality are learned and relearned and performed in ritual interaction. Third, I have shown how, in the case of failed weight-loss surgeries, doctors, patients, and others in the weight-loss surgery community are quick to return to historically premedicalization explanations of weight gain that hinge on familiar understandings of fat people as weak-willed, indulgent, and lazy. I have shown that even as surgeons co-opt and adapt the messages of the fat acceptance movement as they promote weight-loss surgery, they are quick to return to individual designations of patient noncompliance and highly gendered explanations of weight regain and the failure to lose weight after weight-loss surgery. This shift goes largely unquestioned within the broader surgical weight-loss community for reasons I discussed above, such as market interests, patient defensiveness, and cognitive dissonance, as well as the community's focus on success rather than on success and failure. However, all of these reasons are plausible because moral discourses of body size have become so familiar that they are easily drawn upon and employed by patients, doctors, and many others in the weight-loss surgery community and industry to make sense of surgical weight-loss failure without questioning the legitimacy or techniques of biomedicine. That is, the technoscientific intervention was successful, but the patient failed to use it appropriately.

Other scholars (Clarke et al. 2003; Conrad 1992; Conrad and Schneider 1992; Kirkland and Metzl 2010; Sobal 1999, 1995) have emphasized that moral discourses of health, illness, and risk continue to exist even as processes of medicalization and biomedicalization gain prominence. What I have done is to unpack one example of how gendered moral discourses of health continue to hold sway and remain useful even as biomedicine and technoscience expand ever further into the multilayered world of human experience.

This chapter also raises another larger question, namely, How can understanding the case of weight-loss surgery failure add to a theory of the epidemic as a social form since the notion of an epidemic now extends far beyond the realm of mass contagion and death? I hope I have begun to address this question, but it demands an understanding of how discourses of individual responsibility for the success of biomedicine may actually preclude a critique of the viability of technoscientific interventions in an era of postmodern epidemics. If the establishment of a statistical norm such as the BMI is about defining and managing populations, the disciplinary techniques designed to address this population crisis rely on individual behavior.

Much of the construction of or intervention into the obesity epidemic relies on discourses and practices of normative femininity and sexuality. Weight-loss surgery does this too, drawing on the appeal of "normalcy" to return to women's emotionality in explaining weight-loss surgery failure. This ability to return to the cultural figure of the fat woman points to the fact that even as power is increasingly predicated on the self-correction to norms, normalcy itself can never truly be achieved since even those with normal bodies still carry with them the reality or possibility of the inner fat person.

Conclusion

Health at Every Size or Thin at Any Price?

In the years since this research was first conducted, concern over obesity as a social problem has only intensified. The continued search for a miracle weight-loss drug and the expansion of weight-loss surgery eligibility to children and people at lower and lower BMIs has been facilitated by debates about the rising cost of health care, which put obesity front and center. The great recession has brought a new focus on cost cutting, and more and more companies are adopting policies that either offer incentives for weight loss or penalize the overweight and obese. Michelle Obama has chosen childhood obesity as the centerpiece of her agenda as first lady and has declared that we should aim to wipe out childhood obesity in the next decade. Other social and environmental movements, like the slow-food and *locavore* movements, have used social panic about obesity to make the case for their own agendas and, in doing so, have effectively alienated fat people who share their concerns about food production and distribution. In short, concern over obesity and its presumed catastrophic consequences is at the center of national debates around everything from the military to the economy, and obesity has become a rallying point for social causes as varied as environmentalism and education reform.

I develop the concept of a postmodern epidemic to account for the pervasive and flexible place of obesity as a contemporary social problem. A postmodern epidemic is a new social form in which previously unmedicalized phenomenas are framed in terms of the moral panic and chaos characteristic of traditional epidemics of biological contagion and mass death. These postmodern epidemics center on the designation of problematic populations and the universalizing of risk and, at the same time, rely on individual self-correction to norms for their resolution. I argue that, given this shift in the definition of an epidemic, this expands the range of social phenomenas that can be designated as epidemics to the effect that larger issues of social structure and inequality can be reframed in terms of the public and economic threat posed by the deviance of particular individuals, bodies, and populations.

In the case of the obesity epidemic, I have shown that its existence as an epidemic relies on historical understandings of fatness and the need to individualize responsibility for health in an era where state support for public health is low and income and wealth inequality are high. The ascendancy of the BMI as the statistical norm around which the epidemic is centered has facilitated the designation of entire populations as "healthy," "diseased," or "at risk" on the basis of a single number. This power of the BMI to abnormalize more than half of all Americans and to single out children, the poor, and minority populations serves to obscure the social determinants of health. Thus, it becomes useful to a government seeking to minimize spending on social services as well as to an industry seeking to profit from weight-loss efforts. As I showed in chapter I, the agreement of the Department of Health and Human Services (DHHS), the North American Association for the Study of Obesity (NAASO), and the American Obesity Association (AOA) on the designation of obesity as epidemic remained, even as the DHHS sought to individualize both the problem and the solution, while the AOA and NAASO professionalized around efforts to further medicalize obesity and seek government funding for obesity research and surgical and pharmaceutical treatments.

The second main contribution of this book is to show how interventions into the obesity epidemic are based on women's individual attempts to manage the stigma of fatness through normalization projects designed to correct themselves not only to the norm of the BMI, but also, most significantly, to norms of gender, sex, race, and class. Looking at behavioral and surgical weight-loss programs showed that much of people's motivation for weight loss comes from experiencing the social costs of deviating from these norms. In addition, normative constructions of the fat personality and women's inherently abnormal relationship to food and eating also serve to individualize the frequent failure of both behavioral and surgical weight-loss methods. Even as population norms like the BMI and lay and professional discourses about fatness and fat people construct the epidemic, other conventional norms are embedded in its resolution. This is evident because although the epidemic is seen as most rapidly spreading among the poor, minorities, and children, the interventions remain aimed at middle-class white women, those who are already those most likely to attempt to lose weight.

It may seem contradictory that so many resolutions to an epidemic built around panic about the physical and fiscal threat posed by poor, fat minorities would be oriented toward middle-class white women. The usefulness of constructing an epidemic at the population level around individualizing the ill health and poverty of certain populations while at the same time addressing this same epidemic through appealing to the stigma felt by fat white women reveals the dynamism of normalization and the confluence of interests of players at all levels of the epidemic.

While the needs of the government and the public health establishment may be met by defining the obesity epidemic around certain populations, these populations are unlikely to seek out the kinds of behavioral and surgical interventions that have gained popularity in the midst of the epidemic. To be sure, those who seek to promote and profit through weight loss have an interest in calling obesity an epidemic. Participation in groups like Weight Watchers is now tax-deductible, funding for obesity research is at an all-time high, and weight-loss surgeries are increasing exponentially. However, for those interested in selling weight loss, to focus on those populations deemed most problematic would not be particularly profitable given their lower levels of expendable income. Thus, interventions into the epidemic have had to appeal to those with the resources to actually participate in these programs, and they have done that by speaking to the stigma and discrimination felt by fat women. The obesity epidemic is resolved in terms of the individual management of stigma, not concern about health on the part of white, middle-class women.

If the obesity epidemic is constructed and resolved through a confluence of long-standing assumptions about fatness and fat people, the need of government to individualize responsibility for ill health, the interests of the weight-loss industry and professional obesity groups, and norms surrounding sex, gender, race, and class, what, if any, counter-discourses are available to challenge the orthodoxy of the obesity epidemic? Numerous scholars and activists seek to debunk obesity science, highlight discrimination against fat people, and expose the often dangerous profit motives of the diet industry. But scholars and activists have yet to create an alternative framing of weight that is able to successfully quiet or compete with the din of epidemic obesity through research and activism. Nonetheless, they have been able to create a paradigm of weight and health that avoids many of the normative assumptions and interventions I have shown to be at the heart of the obesity epidemic.

The most powerful counter-discourse to that of the "obesity epidemic" comes from the Health at Every Size (HAES) movement.[1] The HAES movement has been around for over twenty-five years, but it has gained renewed vigor in the face of the current panic over epidemic obesity. In general, the HAES paradigm approaches wellness in a way that it is not focused on BMI, weight, or weight loss and embraces diversity in body size. The HAES paradigm recognizes the social determinants of health and advocates for access to quality, nondiscriminatory health care for all as well as access to safe, enjoyable recreation, nutritious food, and leisure time. The HAES paradigm challenges health-care providers to meet the standards of the Hippocratic Oath and "first do no harm" by citing research that shows that dieting can be harmful and often results in weight gain and by doing research on the impact of size discrimination on health.[2] Table 1 presents the main principles and goals of the HAES movement as listed on the website of the Association for Size Diversity and Health (ASDAH).

The HAES community is made up of a nationwide network of health-care professionals, including doctors, nutritionists, nurses, physical therapists, fitness professionals, mental health professionals, and dieticians, as well as activists, medical and academic researchers, educators, parents, lawyers, and others, who seek to offer an alternative perspective, rather than those who take a weight-based approach to health. The HAES community is fairly decentralized and communicates in large part over the Internet, although regional groups do meet and many HAES advocates come together at annual conferences like that of the ASDAH. Though the HAES paradigm does not get even a fraction of the media attention that the

TABLE 1

Health at Every Size Principles and Goals

Principles:

1. Accepting and respecting the diversity of body shapes and sizes

2. Recognizing that health and well-being are multi-dimensional and that they include physical, social, spiritual, occupational, emotional, and intellectual aspects

3. Promoting all aspects of health and well-being for people of all sizes

4. Promoting eating in a manner which balances individual nutritional needs, hunger, satiety, appetite, and pleasure

5. Promoting individually appropriate, enjoyable, life-enhancing physical activity, rather than exercise that is focused on a goal of weight-loss

Long-Term Goals:

1. To develop a forum for discussion, support, and continuing education for professionals who endorse the HAES philosophy

2. To provide information, education, and resources to professionals who are interested in the HAES approach, or who are considering using the HAES approach in their work

3. To promote acceptance of, and respect for, size diversity, and to address cultural and societal issues related to body size and health

4. To facilitate access to quality health care for every individual, regardless of their body size or shape

5. To develop and maintain a website, e-group, and other appropriate on-line resources for on-going communication between ASDAH members

6. To develop a Speaker's Bureau to represent the HAES approach in educational, medical, political, legislative, research, and other appropriate venues

7. To identify qualified HAES representatives to inform, educate, and respond to medical professionals, obesity/weight researchers, and the media

8. To develop and make available resources for implementing HAES in health, fitness, and related industries

9. To develop and maintain resources for review and analysis of health- and weight-related research, in order to encourage scientific literacy and accurate reporting of scientific news

10. To organize a self-supporting annual conference for ASDAH members and supporters to further the mission and goals of the organization

11. To provide policy makers with information and educational resources about the HAES approach and to support public policies that advance the philosophy and goals of HAES

Source: Association for Size Diversity and Health (ASDAH), http://www.bgsu .edu/offices/sa/counseling/page13300.html (accessed January 5, 2012).

obesity epidemic has garnered, HAES-oriented professionals are frequently invited to participate in various forums on weight and health (often in venues hostile to the HAES concept), and for over twenty-five years HAES professionals have published the *Health at Every Size Journal*. The journal offered "research, theory, and practice supporting HAES movement and [was] written to help health professionals understand and practice a compassionate and effective nondieting approach to resolving weight and eating-related concerns."[3]

Beyond public speaking and publishing, advocates engage in a number of other HAES-oriented projects, such as running non-weight-loss-focused exercise classes and HAES-oriented group therapy, blogging, book publishing, developing HAES websites, and even doing weekly HAES radio shows. Though many advocates feel that support for HAES is growing, most also feel that there are many significant barriers to widespread acceptance of the HAES paradigm.

One of the main difficulties in promoting the HAES paradigm is that in the midst of the obesity epidemic, the notion that a fat person could be *fit* or in any way significantly improve his or her health in the absence of weight loss is, in the current climate, simply unthinkable. The most powerful aspect of the obesity epidemic is that it starts from the truism that fatness is, by definition, unhealthy and risky and proceeds without ever questioning that assumption. The taken-for-granted equation of fat with ill health intertwines with and gains legitimacy and cultural intelligibility from other normative discourses of fatness as well as discourses related to gender, sexuality, class, and race. I have shown that even when there is scientific disagreement about the causes and consequences of obesity, these disagreements can be washed over by the general agreement that fat is bad, but also through recourse to other normative discourses.

Time and time again in my research I was confronted with the unthinkability of an orientation toward body size that did not start from the assumption that fatness is unhealthy. Much of my data shows that people's lived experience tells them that the body mass index is not always an accurate measure of health. Indeed, some of the people I observed and spoke with told me that they found the BMI cutoffs to be unreasonable and that they felt healthy if they were a few points or even far more above the current threshold for overweight. Even in the media, there are occasional stories about how women, in particular, should not worry about a "few extra pounds" or stories showcasing "plus-size" celebrities like Queen Latifah, Camryn Mannheim, or Oprah Winfrey and warning about the Hollywood trend toward the super-skinny. While there may be room for a small handful of celebrities who weigh more than the BMI says they should to be accepted as happy, healthy, and attractive people, it is more frequent that the bodies of these celebrities are used to reinforce the idea that while it may be acceptable to be slightly larger than the idealized body, actually being fat is not, and being fat and healthy is even less possible.

As I showed in chapter 2, even when the media present articles that question the rigidity of the BMI or report on the concept that people can be "fat and fit," these articles frequently end with commentary by doctors and obesity researchers who assert that promoting that kind of thinking is dangerous or irresponsible as it may make people think it is alright to be fat if only one eats well and exercises regularly. Moreover, people who consider themselves fat and fit are understood to be making excuses for their fatness and deluding themselves into thinking they could avoid those conditions thought to be associated with obesity without losing considerable amounts of weight.

In my interviews there was a general consensus among members of Weight Watchers and Overeaters Anonymous, as well as among those who had undergone weight-loss surgery, that it is rare, if not impossible, that a fat person could be healthy; and, if they were, they would most certainly not be in the future, although most of my interviewees did not cite health as a prime motivator for losing weight. This promise of future ill health was often used by doctors to convince healthy fat people to choose weight-loss surgery. One of the most interesting examples of the impossibility of the healthy fat person came through my research in Overeaters Anonymous (OA). While my interviewees all seemed to agree that one need not be fat to be a compulsive overeater, if one is fat, then they are, by definition, a compulsive overeater. A striking example of this came in an interview with an OA member when I asked her if it was possible for a woman to weight over 200 pounds and not be a compulsive overeater. This was a potentially awkward moment for my interviewee as I myself weigh something over 200 pounds and I am not a particularly tall person. The woman was quiet for a few moments and thought about my question, and then with a bit of awkward laughter, she said, "I don't see how that could be. I don't see that. My higher power doesn't create bodies to be unhealthy." I followed up by asking her if it is always unhealthy to be fat, to which she responded, "I think for—yes. I think that for most people, if not all, that 250 pounds, that our bodies are not built to carry 250 pounds—they're not built to carry 100 pounds of fat." This exchange is interesting for a number of reasons, but most of all because it illustrates the impossibility of the healthy fat person.

For HAES professionals, in general, and fat HAES professionals, in particular, the cultural unintelligibility of the healthy fat person impacts their credibility and legitimacy as researchers, practitioners, and experts as they are often seen as defensive of their own fatness or as apologists for fat people. As I have shown throughout this book, the visibility of fatness and the long-standing assumptions about the physical and mental deviance of fat people have combined to discredit fat people's experience and expertise as individuals and as professionals. The HAES movement is made up of people of all different sizes, and this size diversity has led many in the movement to notice and discuss the different reception they receive as HAES professionals. In a recent discussion of this topic on a HAES Internet list, one HAES professional, the author of a well-known book questioning the medical orthodoxy surrounding obesity, told of how the book's publisher required him to send in a full-body photo before it would sign a contract to publish the book. In this case, the author happened to be thin, and thus credible in the eyes of the publishers, but as he told the list, it is unlikely that the book ever would have been published if he were fat. One fat nutritionist told of being interviewed for a television newscast and being asked questions primarily about her own weight and eating habits, and not about her expertise as a nutritionist.

One way HAES professionals attempt to mitigate this credibility problem is through presenting and conducting scientific research that supports the claim that BMI in and of itself is not a good measure of health, that fat people can be healthy, and that the correlation between obesity and ill health is often the result of factors, both social and biological, that are masked by an exclusive focus on body weight.[4] Though the spread of the obesity epidemic has opened up a huge flow of research and program money for those trying to contain the epidemic, many people also expressed that it is very difficult to secure funding for research studies that deviate from current obesity orthodoxy. However, some HAES-oriented studies do secure funding; and, in spite of the anti-obesity presentation of findings in traditional obesity research publications, upon closer examination, much traditionally oriented data often yields results that support HAES claims about the actual relationship between weight and health.[5]

One recent example of such research is WomanCare Plus, an ongoing research study affiliated with the Center for Weight and Health at the University of California, Berkeley.[6] A recent article resulting from the study was published in the *International Journal of Obesity* (Amy et al. 2006). The article, titled "Barriers to Routine Gynecological Cancer Screening for White and African-American Obese Women," provides an excellent example of HAES-oriented research because it takes an oft-cited correlation between obesity and gynecological cancer and questions the validity of a sole focus on BMI by showing other factors that may explain much of this correlation. According to the study, increased morbidity and mortality from gynecological cancers is often cited by obesity researchers as one of the many health risks faced by obese women, yet it is also the case that fat women are less likely than thinner women to get routine screening for these cancers, many of which are curable if diagnosed and treated early.[7] Thus, the authors do not question the correlation between higher BMI values and the prevalence of these types of cancer; rather, they provide an explanation for this correlation that goes beyond a simple equation of fatness with ill health and risk.

The WomanCare Plus study seeks to understand the factors that contribute to this lower screening rate. The study surveyed 498 white and African American women with BMIs between 25 (the current cutoff for overweight) and 122 about their history of gynecological cancer screenings as well as what, if anything, had prevented them from getting such screenings. The study found that significant differences in screening rates between women with BMIs less than 25 and those with BMIs higher than 25 remained even when adjusting for age, education, race, and health insurance access. Indeed, though many fat people have difficulty getting health insurance, over 90 percent of the women in the WomanCare Plus study had health insurance. The main finding of this study, thus far, is that obese women report that they delay cancer-screening tests and that they feel their weight is a barrier to getting good health care. The study also reports that as BMI increased, so too did the number of women who reported delaying screenings (Amy et al. 2006).

When asked if they had ever delayed seeking health care or cancer screening because of their weight, fully 41 percent of the women in the study reported that they had. The study also found that the number of women who delayed care was significantly higher among women with a BMI greater than or equal to 55. Of the women in this BMI group, 68 percent reported delaying care and 83 percent felt that their weight was a barrier to getting appropriate health care (Amy et al. 2006). While the reported delays were associated with BMI, they were not significantly related to age, education level, insurance coverage, or type of health coverage (private, HMO, or health clinic). In addition, 73 percent of the women in the study cited one or more weight-related barriers to health care. The most frequently cited weight-related barriers to care are shown in table 2.

The study also found that women with higher BMIs were more likely to experience these barriers. Perhaps one of the most interesting findings of the study is that woman who delayed care were also significantly more likely to have dieted five or more times, compared with women who did not delay care (41 percent and 25 percent, respectively). Though the authors do not speculate as to why there is this difference between those who had been on five or more diets and those who had not, their study does bring into question the assumption that dieting for weight loss

---

TABLE 2

WomanCare Plus: Weight-Related Barriers to Health Care

- Disrespectful treatment (36%)
- Embarrassment about being weighed (35%)
- Negative attitudes of providers (36%)
- Advice to lose weight, even if unrelated to your medical condition (46%)
- Small gowns, exam tables, and equipment (46%)

Source: Amy et al. 2006, 147–55.

improves health status among obese women both because diets typically
fail and often result in weight gain over time (Bacon 2008; Gaesser 2002)
and because one of the greatest predictors of cancer survival is early
detection and treatment. This finding also suggests that recent government recommendations that physicians weigh all patients at each visit
and discuss weight loss, diet, and exercise with those whose BMI values
categorize them as overweight or obese may be misguided and perhaps
even indirectly have negative health-related consequences for their heavier
patients.

Studies like WomanCare Plus are important for a number of reasons.
First and foremost, they do not start with the assumption that obesity and
overweight have an inherent negative impact on overall health; indeed,
some HAES researchers (Ernsberger and Haskew 1987) have even found
positive health outcomes associated with overweight and obesity. Second,
HAES researchers also do not start with the assumption that there are no
health problems associated with higher than average weights, but they do
seek to provide a more complex interrogation and analysis of correlations
between higher than average weights and certain conditions that do not
start and end with the body mass index. Indeed, the WomanCare Plus study
points out that we can't actually know what, if any, association there is
between BMI and higher gynecological cancer rates until we understand
the impact of size discrimination on women's ability and willingness to get
screened at the recommended intervals and using appropriate equipment.[8]
Third, HAES-informed research moves beyond individualized explanations
for ill health that are characteristic of the obesity epidemic and earlier
discourses of fatness since it views health as an outcome of social as well as
biological and behavioral processes. Finally, as with the HAES movement
in general, HAES researchers appear to have a broader understanding of
health in which health-promoting interventions are not necessarily
designed to push people toward a single state of perfect health and a
single, limited range of acceptable body size, but where health is an ongoing process, and being *healthy* or *healthier* is not the same for everyone.

Of course, in an era where health status has become a measure of
moral status, there is no such thing as pure resistance, and the Health at
Every Size paradigm and the fat and fit movement have been criticized by
some as being yet another incarnation of a moral imperative to be healthy.

As early as the 1980s, some fat activists saw the fat and fit discourse as playing into a national obsession with fitness. In an essay written for a fat-positive newsletter, Karen Stimson (1983) questioned the efficacy and political implications of the growing fat and fit discourse within the fat liberation movement. Stimson suggested that, at first blush, the fat and fit approach seemed reasonable because, contrary to popular belief, fat people can be active and healthy without losing weight and because encouraging and facilitating exercise is important for everyone. Citing fat athletes and dancers who confirm the potential fitness of fat people, Stimson went on to question and offer an explanation for the timing of the fat acceptance movement's embracing of the fat and fit concept: "So, why are we making a big fuss over this in the movement right now? Partly, I suspect, because we are trying to change our image from the 'fat slob' stereotype to something more positive. We see embracing fitness for fat people as a way of accomplishing this goal" (1983). Stimson suggested that this approach to fat oppression is dangerous, elitist, and, in the end, unlikely to truly change stereotypes about fat people. She warned, "It is important that as a movement we do NOT adopt elitist attitudes which tend to weed out the very people most in need of what we claim to support" (1983).

For Stimson, there is a key distinction between advocating for people of all sizes to have access to the leisure time and resources to be physically fit and basing the movement's claim to civil rights for fat people on them becoming fit. She suggested that any acceptance that fat people gain on the basis of being "fit" is tenuous at best and likely to backfire politically: "Fat people have been collectively victimized by healthism. We must be careful not to use it against ourselves. . . . The idea that any of us is somehow 'better' than 'those other fat people' because we dress in designer jeans, or eat 'health foods,' or work out at the gym every day, is political poison" (1983). Stimson went on to say that this view is particularly insidious because "this subtle sense of superiority is so easily incorporated into our rising self esteem when we become politically aware" (1983).

This concern for the normative potential of the fat and fit and the HAES perspectives remains a consideration among many contemporary fat activists, though this unease often goes unspoken within the HAES community. I recently brought up the topic on a list serve of HAES professionals of which I am a member, and the responses indicated that health moralism is a real concern for many people who are very dedicated to promoting the HAES paradigm. In fact, several people expressed relief that I had broached the topic since they, too, had been thinking about the same issue. One list member said that in certain settings where he is in discussions and debates with medical professionals, he finds himself using the fat and fit argument in a way that implies that these fat people are *better* than those fat people who have health problems. He expressed frustrations and asked for others' thoughts: "How do we address 'but it's just not healthy to be fat' without getting caught up in 'fit and fat'?" This appears to be a fine line for many HAES advocates and fat activists. They feel that they want to make the important point that fat people can be and often are just as healthy, if not more so, than thinner people, but they do not want to lapse into their own version of health moralism.

Through tracing key moments in the construction of the obesity epidemic and linking this to the experience of people trying to lose or control their weight, this book has shown that, now more than ever, normative constructions of race, class, gender, sexuality, and health are centered on the identification and normalization of both deviant and potentially deviant bodies. With the proliferation of postmodern epidemics like obesity, it is critical to understand how these norms inform and construct our notions of health and risk. As the above discussion of the HAES paradigm shows, in an era of heightened health morality, there is no perfect counterdiscourse to counter that of the obesity epidemic or other epidemics of normalization. However, the discussion of the HAES paradigm does show that there are significant ways in which research and activism can again bring attention to structural barriers to health as well as to the economic and political utility—for various, vested interests—of framing social phenomena as "epidemics" in an era of declining social support.

APPENDIX: METHODOLOGY

In a general sense, the methodology of this book is based on Michel Foucault's concept of "genealogy." Genealogy, for Foucault (1977), is a way of understanding history that abandons the search for origins and meta-historical truths. Rather than searching for the linear truth of history, genealogy concerns itself with tracing what has become repeated and naturalized in history and with phenomenas viewed as natural and eternal; it also must concern itself with what was absent, what could not be said, and what might have been and wasn't. I see this book as a partial genealogy of the obesity epidemic.

I say "partial" for two reasons. First, because I believe that given the abandonment of the search for a meta-narrative, coupled with the ever-shifting nature of modern power and the relations of knowledge, any genealogy is, by definition, partial. My second reason is perhaps more practical; to offer a more complete genealogy of the obesity epidemic is far beyond the scope of what can be realistically accomplished in a project of this size.

What I have done in this book is to offer a genealogy of certain moments, aspects, and discourses of the obesity epidemic in the hope of bringing to light the naturalized assumptions of truth upon which its construction relies as well as show how these assumptions are of consequence in the normalizing techniques that have arisen as treatments for the "obesity epidemic." Attention to the relationship between language and power is critical to understanding the material and individual consequences of the interaction of various discourses. I also follow from Dawne Moon in arguing that this attention to language and power tells us "how socially informed ways of looking at the world can come to seem natural and timeless and how this appearance of timelessness can guide and foreclose possibilities" (2004, 9).

The data presented were gathered through the use of three methods: textual analysis, participant observation, and in-depth interviewing. Given the focus on public policy and media in chapters 1 and 2 of the book, that section is weighted heavily toward textual analysis. The more interactional and experiential quality of the interventions, such as Weight Watchers and Overeaters Anonymous, which I highlight in the later empirical chapters, necessitates greater attention to the relationship between power/knowledge and the lived experience and social relations of individuals and groups. Scholars following in post-structural and Foucauldian traditions tend to emphasize the importance of text, and in my use of text, I am no exception.

Yet as Moon (2004) rightly points out, this nearly exclusive focus on text is problematic when studying non-hierarchical systems of power as printed text already bears the mark of hierarchy and leaves out those whose experiences are not preserved in text of one form or another. Thus, in chapters 3 and 4, I use participant observation and in-depth interviews to better understand how people make sense of the language of the obesity epidemic and naturalized knowledges about the body, gender, sexuality, class, and race that inform it, as well as how people negotiate these knowledges in confronting their own experience with the stigma of overweight.[1]

In chapter 1, I use data from three Department of Health and Human Services (DHHS) *Healthy People* reports: *Healthy People, Healthy People 2000*, and *Healthy People 2010*. I selected this series of reports not because they offer a comprehensive picture of the public health community's orientation toward overweight and obesity, but because they represent an ongoing effort by the DHHS to identify national public health priorities and goals and to outline and track the progress of specific public health objectives. I also chose this series of reports because of the controversy surrounding the place of overweight and obesity in *Healthy People 2010*. This debate opened a window through which I could see competing discourses of weight at work as well as understand critical points of convergence and divergence between the public health community and the American Obesity Association (AOA) and the North American Association for the Study of Obesity (NAASO).

In addition to the three *Healthy People* reports, I analyze a DHHS (1998) report entitled *Leading Indicators for Healthy People 2010* and three later reports from the Institutes of Medicine (1999b, 1999a, 1998) Committee on Leading Health Indicators for Healthy People 2010. I also use documents related to *Healthy People 2010* found on the websites of NAASO and AOA, including the AOA's publication, *Healthy Weight 2010*.

Chapter 2, on the media construction of the epidemic, draws from 751 articles on obesity that appeared in the *New York Times* between 1990 and 2001 in order to identify the main themes and trace the contours of the epidemic.[2] I focus most closely on a series of articles on the "fat epidemic," published in the fall of 2000. I treat these articles as social constructions and not as social facts. Thus, these articles represent the media construction of an epidemic, and not objective information on science or medicine. Using textual analysis, I identified three dominant themes in these articles—chaos and containment, professionalization of common sense, and nature and culture. These three sets of linked categories help elucidate the basic social processes central to the construction of the epidemic. They also reflect pairings that arise in various ways within the social scientific literature on epidemics, medical sociology, and feminist theory (Conrad 1992). An analysis of these categories, which are typically seen as oppositional, highlights the tension, contradictions, and contested nature of this epidemic.

The *New York Times* reporting on obesity does not represent a comprehensive picture of the media's approach to the epidemic. However, I have chosen the *Times* as my main data source for three reasons. First, the obesity epidemic has been portrayed as a national crisis of major significance, and it is only fitting that a study of the media construction of this epidemic should rely on a leading national news source. In addition, the *Times* occupies a privileged place as a leading opinion center and trend setter among intellectuals, professionals, and policy makers (Gitlin 1980). Second, the *Times* is particularly noted for its science writing, and many of the contradictions and complexities of this epidemic orbit around perceptions of science and medicine. Third, as medical and scientific knowledge is no longer primarily transmitted within the doctor-patient relation, but through democratization of access to this knowledge via the media and the Internet, sources like the *Times* become more central to the layperson's understanding of health, science, and medicine (Clarke et al. 2003).

The data presented in chapter 3 on Weight Watchers and Overeaters Anonymous was collected through three primary methods: participant observation; in-depth, semi-structured interviews; and textual analysis. I conducted interviews with fifteen active Weight Watchers members and fourteen active Overeaters Anonymous members.[3] Interviewees were recruited via a posting on an online community bulletin board and, in the case of Overeaters Anonymous members, through a snowball sample. In addition to these interviews, I conducted participant observation in a twelve-week course of the Weight Watchers program and attended twenty-two Overeaters Anonymous meetings. I also observed an Overeaters Anonymous list serve of over five hundred members for over a year. This list is not run by Overeaters Anonymous but is organized around the principles of Overeaters Anonymous and the twelve steps. I have also included data from a close reading of both Overeaters Anonymous and Weight Watchers literature.

While I observed a Weight Watchers list serve for a short time, I chose not to include data from those observations in this chapter for two main reasons. First, the Weight Watchers website is, first and foremost, a source of information about the program. The content of the messages on the Weight Watchers list serve most often revolves around questions about point values of certain foods and the exchange of recipes. In order to access these discussion boards, recipes, and other features, members must purchase a paid monthly subscription. Second, at that time in Weight Watchers, list serves did not play such a central role in members' participation in the program as a whole as they do in Overeaters Anonymous. For many Overeaters Anonymous members, the list serve is their primary mode of participation in the program as it offers a twenty-four-hour network of other members. Given the requirements of weigh-ins at Weight Watchers, the message boards and list serves are a supplement and, according to the people I interviewed, not very central to their experience of the program at the time.

Over the course of six months in 2002 and 2003, I attended twenty-two Overeaters Anonymous meetings in northern California. The meetings I attended were held in a variety of locations, most often churches, but I also attended meetings at a community center, a hospital, and a YMCA conference room. All of the meetings I attended were open to the public.[4]

I attended meetings at various times of day, finding the evening and week-end meetings to be the largest. While all Overeaters Anonymous meetings follow the same basic format, the focus of the meetings varies widely. Some of the meetings are focused on studying the twelve steps, some on reading other Overeaters Anonymous literature, and others orbit around issues specific to certain groups of people, like lesbians and gays, those who have lost or want to lose at least one hundred pounds, women, or young people. Though they may have a specific focus, in general, these meetings remain open to the public.

Chapter 4, on weight-loss surgery, draws on data from three primary sources. First, ethnographic data were derived from participant observation in eleven weight-loss surgery informational seminars, seven support-group meetings, a weekend-long national convention of the group Obesity Help, and two years of observation of a variety of online message boards and chat rooms for those who have had or are interested in weight-loss surgery.

Second, I conducted ten in-depth, semi-structured interviews with post-operative weight-loss surgery patients. My interviewees were comprised of one man and nine women ranging in age from twenty-seven to fifty-four. All interviewees were between three months and three years post-operative. All had the Roux-en-Y (RNY) gastric bypass, with the exception of one interviewee who had a different and less common procedure. One of my interviewees identified herself as Latina, and two as African American; the rest identified as white. Interviewees were from both rural and urban areas of northern California. Interviewees were recruited through interview requests placed on weight-loss surgery and community message boards as well as through a snowball sample.

Finally, I did a textual analysis of informational literature from a variety of weight-loss surgery programs and *Obesity Help Magazine*.[5] Program literature represents those programs whose informational seminars I attended as well as literature present at the Obesity Help convention.

Bringing these three methods together provides a context for the epidemic and a depth of analysis that any one alone could not have achieved. This is particularly true as it pertains to understanding the experience of people, a topic that has been left out of most social, scientific analyses of the obesity crisis. Thus, using textual, interview, and observational data serves to bridge the gap between analyses of the obesity epidemic that focus on its history and construction in the media, in policy circles, and in the medical literature and those analyses that focus on the lives and experiences of fat people and others confronted with a culture in which so much moral valuation is put on body size.

Given the face-to-face nature of in-depth interviewing and participant observation, it makes sense to ask about an author's own relationship to a research topic. In this case, I suspect readers will wonder about my weight and if and how it impacted my orientation to the topic of obesity and my relationship to the people I was studying. In the parlance of the obesity epidemic, I would, indeed, be considered obese, morbidly so by current measures. Along with my training as a sociologist, this gives me a perspective on obesity and the link between weight and health that could be generally described as critical. In this book I have been careful not to make any claims about the "true" relationship between weight and health even as I have critiqued the language of obesity and the techniques used to *cure* it. Nonetheless, given the entrenched nature of what we think we know about weight, health, and fat people, my own size will likely garner accusations that I am being defensive or that my motivations for writing the book are purely political. To this I would say that to the extent that the personal is political, and to the extent that allowing marginalized people's words and experiences to shed light on the claims and motivations of the powerful, this is a political book; it could scarcely not be. On the other hand, I have been rigorous in my methodology, and I have grounded my analysis in scholarly literature in a way that makes my claims far more academic than personal.

Those who study marginalized groups, as I would argue fat people in America are, have long debated who is best suited to study these groups, insiders or outsiders (Mehra 2008; Merton 1972). In the case of this book, I feel that my own size was an advantage in interviewing other fat people and in observing in settings like Weight Watchers and Overeaters Anonymous meetings, where weight is central to the groups' activity. I was never questioned about my presence in settings like public weight-loss surgery seminars, where I might have stood out at a smaller size; and in settings where my role as observer was more overt, I was welcomed in a way that I might not have been if I had not been seen as engaged in a similar struggle with weight. In interviews, I felt that interviewees trusted me more than they would have trusted a researcher of more average size. My own size gave people a sense of common cause with me, and they assumed a shared experience that was often right on target. On the other hand, I was never dishonest with an interviewee who asked about my own weight-loss attempts or eating habits. I simply told them that, while I have made peace with my body and no longer attempt to change my size, I, too, spent years engaged in a struggle with self-hatred and failed weight-loss efforts.

In short, as I have argued throughout the book, weight has become both an outward sign of health and a marker of the inner state of the soul. While fat people may be the most obviously impacted by this current, dominant cultural equation of weight with both health and morality, this is a situation from which no one is exempt. The obesity epidemic is not simply about fat people, it is about risk, citizenship, gender, race, class, sexuality, morality, and the list goes on. The point is that we are all impli-cated in the obesity epidemic; and thus, anyone trying to research this topic would come to the task with a body that would be read by research subjects and book readers alike for its relationship to current understand-ings of size and its relationship to a whole host of other social categories and meanings.

NOTES

INTRODUCTION

1. There are several recent books that do take on the science of obesity. See Bacon 2008; Campos 2004; Gaesser 2002; Oliver 2006.

2. Graham was not the only popular health reformer in this time period. Horace Fletcher's more scientific method of "Fletcherizing," or chewing, food also gained popularity around the 1830s (Schwartz 1986).

3. As many have pointed out (Bordo 1993; Chang and Christakis 2002; Stearns 1997), before the turn of the century, and in times of scarcity, larger bodies were seen as robust and healthy. However, Graham's concern with food purity and his equation of a person's dietary habits with his or her moral standing presages some of the language used by today's organic and slow-food movements.

4. The exact formula for calculating BMI is weight (in kilograms) divided by height (in meters) squared. For a more detailed history of the BMI and other measures of calculating overweight see Oliver 2006.

5. Many, though not all, people working in the Health at Every Size (HAES) paradigm have their roots in the "fat acceptance movement." The general purpose of the fat acceptance and fat liberation movements is activism and education against size discrimination. Movement activists believe that rigid Western beauty standards, especially for women, a $60-billion-a-year American diet industry, and a medical profession influenced by both have re-created a society in which fat people are alienated, discriminated against, stigmatized, and deemed morally flawed. It is the movement's assertion that—because dominant U.S. beliefs falsely deem fatness as necessarily unhealthy, the result of individual deviance, and entirely changeable—size discrimination has not been widely problematized. Within these movements, considerable attention has been paid to how to deal with the increasing discrimination and stigma experienced by fat people as a result of the obesity epidemic and the ostensible concern for the health of fat people.

6. For a more detailed discussion of method and methodology, see the appendix.

CHAPTER 1   OBESITY AS A "LEADING HEALTH INDICATOR"

1. The U.S. Department of Health, Education, and Welfare is now known as the U.S. Department of Health and Human Services (DHHS).

2. This shift is in line with that noted by many medical historians and medical sociologists (Clarke et al. 2003; Conrad and Schneider 1992; Lupton 1996; Rose 1994; Starr 1984; Turner 1994).

3. Interestingly, much of the attention to weight in the first two *Healthy People* reports focuses on underweight, particularly, low-birth-weight babies and women who do not gain sufficient weight during pregnancy. Underweight related to eating disorders like anorexia and bulimia is mentioned once in *Healthy People 2000*. The goals in the first *Healthy People* report are far less detailed than those in the subsequent two reports. This is likely a result of a lack of baseline data to set specific target goals. Thus, in *Healthy People 2000* the aim is general "weight reduction" and does not include a specific population goal, as do the later reports.

4. It is interesting that this measure shows the rate of obesity in poor men as being less than half that of men above the poverty line though obesity was already more prevalent in poorer women. This could be indicative of several factors: higher rates of smoking among poorer men, the more physical nature of blue-collar jobs in the 1960s and 1970s than in the present, as well as even less stringent expectations of body size among non-poor men than those that exist today.

5. As the reports set ten-year health goals, the titles of the reports include the goal date in their title. Thus, *Healthy People 2000* was first published in 1990, and the original *Healthy People* report containing the goals for 1990 was published in 1979.

6. There is, however, an appendix to the full report that compiles objectives and promises increased collection of data that are of particular significance for specific racial and ethnic minority groups, the elderly, and the disabled. Of course, increased attention to the health challenges of various minority groups also allows them to become targets for intervention, and obesity is no exception to this trend. Blaming the "cultural practices" (hygiene, dietary, and child-rearing practices among them) of specific populations for the emergence and spread of epidemic disease is not a new phenomenon and offers a linkage between the discourses of culture in both traditional and postmodern epidemics (Craddock 1995; Dew 1999; Hatty and Hatty 1999; Rosenberg 1962; Treichler 1999).

7. Most of the consortium is made up of groups that have professionalized around specific health issues, commercial interests, or social issues. This includes groups as diverse as the American College of Health Care Executives, the Sugar Association, Mothers Against Drunk Driving, the American Medical Association, and the American Obesity Association. As I show in my discussion of the leading health indicators in the *Healthy People 2010* report, the confluence of interests between many of these consortium members and the interests of

the public health establishment had a significant impact on the emergence of obesity as a twenty-first-century epidemic that is nonetheless framed very differently based on the needs and interests of different groups.

8. It should be noted that many objectives are cross-listed in multiple priority areas; thus, these objectives actually appear six times in the report, making 6 out of 332 total objectives that explicitly mention overweight or obesity.

9. As I discussed in the introduction, in 1998, the BMI threshold for "overweight" would be decreased to 25 for all people regardless of sex or body fat composition, thus greatly increasing the number of Americans falling into both categories of "overweight" and "obese" by the time the 2010 objectives were written.

10. I discuss the development of these LHIs in greater detail later.

11. As with the objectives in *Healthy People 2000*, those in *Healthy People 2010* are also cross-listed in other focus areas. For example, objectives 19–1 and 19–2 are cross-listed without modification in the focus areas on heart disease and diabetes. The three objectives are stated exactly as they are printed in the *Healthy People 2010*, but it should be noted that each objective is also accompanied by a chart breaking down the bascline and targets by sub-categories of gender, race and ethnicity, age, family income level, disability status, and "special populations," which include people with and without arthritis, with and without diabetes, and with and without high blood pressure.

12. In the case of children and adolescents, DHHS uses a measure of overweight and obesity defined as at or above the age and gender specific ninety-fifth percentile of BMI, based on the revised CDC (Centers for Disease Control) Growth Charts for the United States. Even those most committed to using the BMI as the sole indicator of overweight and obesity recognize that given the variation of growth rates in children and adolescents, use of a specific BMI cutoff in these populations is an unreliable measure. Most, like DHHS, use a percentile-based measure for children and adolescents. It is important to note that while perhaps a better measure of relative size than the use of adult BMI cutoff points, defining childhood obesity as any BMI above the age- and gender-specific 95th percentile guarantees that regardless of actual weights, the percentage of children and adolescents in the "obese" category will remain relatively stable.

13. Prior to 1998 American BMI values had set a BMI of 27.8 as the point at which people were diagnosed as overweight.

14. A more complete genealogy of the BMI itself is needed. Such a study would and should consider at greater length what other measures of overweight and obesity, as well as the relationship between weight and health, have been proposed, developed, partially developed, or discarded to allow for the BMI to be established as the only widely accepted measure of body weight.

15. The Centers for Disease Control and Prevention (CDCP) estimates the annual cost of obesity for the year 2002 to have been approximately 92 billion dollars. These oft-cited costs of obesity have continued to skyrocket.

16. The report notes that the exception to this general lack of interest in the life-stage goals of *Healthy People* was the substantial national attention paid to the issue of infant mortality.

17. The North American Society for the Study of Obesity (NAASO) was an organization of obesity researchers. In 2007, it merged with the American Obesity Association (AOA) to become one organization, the Obesity Society.

18. The American Obesity Association website was removed after it merged with NAASO. The new website states that the mission of the Obesity Society is this: "through research, education, and advocacy, to better understand, prevent, and treat obesity and improve the lives of those affected." (See http://www .obesity.org/about-us/mission-and-vision.htm for the full statement of vision, mission, and values.)

19. The AOA had a more varied and, thus, larger membership base than NAASO. AOA memberships ranged from $15 per year for individuals to $1,000 per year for some organizations.

20. As noted, the old AOA website content was replaced when AOA and NAASO merged. The quote cited is from the old website.

21. See note 20, this quote is from the old AOA website.

22. Ibid.

23. The former website, http://www.naaso.org, has been replaced with the merged website http://obesity.org. Quote cited is from the older website.

24. See note 23, this quote is from the now defunct NAASO website, http://www .naaso.org.

25. Ibid.

26. Ibid.

27. This report figured prominently on the AOA website for several years under the page heading "AOA Comments to the U.S. Department of Health and Human Services: Recognition of Obesity in the U.S. Health Charter, Healthy People 2010. December 1998" but is no longer available online.

28. In section two of their report, the AOA offers a listing of thirty-four conditions for which obesity is "an independent risk factor or an aggravating agent." This list includes conditions that are commonly associated with obesity in the media and public health circles as well as some less frequently heard conditions, including breast cancer in men, cancer of the esophagus, impaired immune response, urinary stress incontinence, and traumatic injuries to teeth.

CHAPTER 2   ALL THE NEWS THAT'S *FAT* TO PRINT

1. I have chosen to focus my analysis in this chapter on the *New York Times* for three reasons. First, the obesity epidemic has been portrayed as a national crisis of major significance, and it is only fitting that a study of this epidemic should rely on a leading national news source. The *Times* occupies a privileged

place as a leading opinion center and setter among intellectuals, professionals, policy makers, and the general educated public (Gitlin 1980). Second, the *Times* is noted for its science writing, and many of the contradictions and complexities of this epidemic orbit around perceptions of science and medicine. Third, as medical and scientific knowledge is no longer primarily transmitted within the doctor-patient relationship, but through "democratization" of access to health-related information via the media and the Internet, sources like the *Times* become more central to the layperson's understanding of health, science, and medicine (Barker 2005; Clarke et al. 2003; Conrad 2007).

2. Number of articles was based on searches in Lexis-Nexis.

3. The entire "Fat Epidemic" series can be accessed at http://www.nytimes.com/library/national/science/health/obesity-health.html.

4. Beyond their work in the *Times,* both Jane Brody and Gina Kolata have published multiple books on the topics of health, weight, and nutrition (Brody 1980, 2000a; Kolata 2003, 2008).

5. Since the early 1980s, with the publication of the fat activist collection *Shadow on a Tightrope* (Shoenfielder and Weiser 1983), there has been a steady body of work coming from fat activists and their allies questioning fat discrimination, the science of obesity, and the diet industry. However, until recently, these works have failed to gain national attention outside of the activist community.

6. BMI is calculated by dividing weight (in kilograms) by height (in meters) squared. See NHLBI at http://www.nhlbi.nih.gov/index.html for more information on BMI calculation and how it is presented for public usage. The website includes a BMI calculator.

7. As I have discussed earlier, the significance of calculating the "cost" of obesity comes not from the actual dollar amount given, but in the association of such an "individual" problem with such astronomical public costs.

8. For a more recent critique of the BMI, see http://www.npr.org/templates/story/story.php?storyId=106268439. This type of fetishization of the cultural origins of epidemics is not unique to obesity. As Paula Lantz and Karen Booth (1998) point out in their study of the breast cancer epidemic, though increases in breast cancer rates in the 1980s can largely be explained by increased use of mammography and early screening, this is obscured by a focus on the purported pathological repercussions of women's changing social roles.

9. Indeed, many critics of the obesity epidemic have pointed out that behaviors that are seen as indicative of eating disorders in those who are thin are often precisely the sorts of behaviors that are prescribed for those who are of higher weights (Boero and Pascoe forthcoming; Pascoe and Boero forthcoming; Thomas and Wilkerson 2005; Wann 1998).

10. In February 2011, the criteria for lap band devices was expanded to include those with a BMI of 35 or higher with no co-morbid condition and 30 or higher with at least one co-morbid condition. See the FDA's website (http://www.fda

.gov/MedicalDevices/ProductsandMedicalProcedures/DeviceApprovalsand Clearances/Recently-ApprovedDevices/ucm248133.htm) for more information on this device and the approval of the expanded criteria. This expansion effectively opened the market for lap band devices from 15 million to over 41 million Americans.

11. American Society of Metabolic and Bariatric Surgeons (ASMBS) was known as the American Society of Bariatric Surgeons (ASBS) until 2008. Figures quoted here are from earlier items on its website. The organization provides the latest figures and other position papers in their "Media" section on its website: http://www.asmbs.org/Newsite07/resources/asmbs_items.htm. It is interesting to note the recent adding of the word "Metabolic" to its name and rhetoric. Recent studies have shown evidence that some bariatric surgeries may help reduce glucose levels and type 2 diabetes and have led some surgeons to push for a change in the name and focus (see http://www.cornellsurgery.org/pro/services/gi-metabolic/ as an example). This represents an expansion of their potential market and strengthens their assertion that the surgery is a useful intervention and is addressing a serious problem.

12. The Obesity Society (http://obesity.org) is a merger of two groups, the American Obesity Association (AOA) and the North American Association for the Study of Obesity (NAASO). According to its website, the purpose of this group is to be "a community of professionals dedicated to researching, preventing and treating obesity." The Obesity Society has strongly advocated, both in its previous forms and in its merged entity, that obesity is a disease. See chapter 1 for a full discussion of this position.

13. The Institute of Medicine (IOM) is a private, nonprofit organization chartered by Congress that advises the federal government on health policy.

14. In this section I move beyond an exclusive analysis of data from the *Times* to discuss the release of two policy reports on obesity, both of which received significant coverage in the *Times*.

15. See the "About IOM" section of its website for a full description of its mission and work (http://www.iom.edu/About-IOM.aspx).

16. The entire National Academies of Science press release of December 6, 1994, is available online at http://www8.nationalacademies.org/onpinews/newsitem .aspx?RecordID=11514.

17. Throughout all of the articles I reviewed, there is almost always a paragraph that restates the need for diet and exercise in order to lose weight, even when studies are cited that suggest everything from viruses and social contact to specific genes are implicated in obesity. This is very similar to something Paul Campos (2004, 45) noted: "Despite their own article's evidence, the authors will conclude that 'overweight' people . . . should diet anyway. Such conclusions, [Susan] Wooley says, can be interpreted as a coded message to the diet and drug industry: 'P.S. Fund me again.'" I would submit that both the researcher being interviewed who accepts funding and the newspaper that accepts advertising

from these industries feel compelled to not rock the boat of the traditionally acceptable advice that no weight loss will occur without diet and exercise, and no diet and exercise will occur without willpower.

18. This represents a shift from the type of medicalization of knowledge in which women's knowledge is undercut and delegitimated by the rise of science and medicine (Ehrenreich and English 1978; Martin 1987).

19. This idea that fat is the cultural realization of genetic potential is a common way of circumventing the nature-culture debate over the origins of fatness.

20. "Asian," in these articles, generally refers only to the Japanese and Chinese.

21. The relationship between culture and the individual is a dynamic one. Were it not constructed as a binary within these articles, we might not see such an overwhelming focus on individual solutions to social problems. My point is not to prescribe social rather than individual action vis-à-vis obesity; indeed, it is not to prescribe any action at all. Rather, my point is that when the problem is located within an individual who appears to be a rational actor outside of cultural and structural constraints, there are particular consequences, namely, an exclusive focus on individual "cures" to social problems.

22. I will return to more recent reporting on obesity in the conclusion.

CHAPTER 3   NORMATIVE PATHOLOGY AND UNIQUE DISEASE

1. The former Duchess of York is a longtime Weight Watchers spokesperson.

2. The free food journals that are given out each week are small, folded booklets that contain space for recording one's daily food intake.

3. Although Weight Watchers does not calculate specific BMI values for each client, its ranges are based on the ranges provided by the BMI.

4. This is according to Weight Watcher's own market research and is cited on their website, http://www.weightwatchersinternational.com. It was not independently confirmed.

5. Throughout her book, Nidetch maintains that there are core personality differences between fat people and thin people. She portrays fat people as selfish, lazy, stupid, dishonest, and, alternately, funny, social, and personable. Either way, any personality trait of fat people is either an expression of their inner self-hatred or an attempt to mask that same self-hatred. Others (Bordo 1993; Thomas and Wilkerson 2005) have explored the meaning of this framing of the fat, particularly female, personality. The distinctions between personalities of people of different sizes in Weight Watchers today is far less rigid; but, in general, and as I will show in the next chapter on bariatric surgery, this "commonsense" understanding of the fat personality and subjectivity continues to have a profound impact on how programs present themselves and frame the success or failure of their participants.

6. For a more detailed discussion of the history of various Weight Watchers' food plans, see Stinson (2001).

7. As Spitzack (1990) reminds us, for Foucault, the act of "confessing" or talking about one's transgressions not only confirms the deviance of those transgressions, but is central to the normalizing process of those who confess. "Speaking the truth about one's self . . . underscores the power of normative bases of judgment, for implicit in the act of confession is a promise to realign thoughts and actions with predominant social values" (Spitzack 1990). In Weight Watchers, this confession at once confirms the deviance of women's relationship to food and weight while also providing evidence of the speaker's desire to normalize, insofar as possible, her behavior, body, and self.

8. In Weight Watchers a lifetime member is one who has stayed within two pounds above or below his or her goal weight for longer than two months. Lifetime members are given free entrance to meetings, and to maintain lifetime status, they must also attend at least one meeting per month to weigh in. This arrangement serves the dual purpose of helping members maintain notoriously short-lived weight losses as well as guaranteeing that newer members are likely to come in to contact with one or more examples of program success at any given meeting (Stinson 2001).

9. The Weight Watchers program is ever changing, so the descriptions of the program in this work reflect the program as it was in the fall of 2002 and winter of 2003.

10. The subtle ways in which members can sabotage themselves are often referenced in meetings, presumably to remind members that if they gain weight or fail to lose any, it is most likely because they are not following the program properly.

11. The term *balanced nutrition* is a contested one. Though Weight Watchers generally recommends a balance like that represented in the FDA's food pyramid, the oft-changing history of what is considered sound nutrition and recent debates over the nature of carbohydrates and refined sugars, fats, and protein have shed light on the political and economic forces that often play a significant role in debates over what and how much people need to eat.

12. Lifetime members must continue to weigh in once a month to maintain their lifetime status. This presumably serves two purposes. First, it keeps members involved in the program and may improve their chances of keeping lost weight off. Second, the presence at meetings of people who have achieved and maintained their goal weights may serve as a motivation to newcomers and members who have not yet "made goal."

13. The group journal is a journal that is passed to a new volunteer each week. At the following meeting the person who had the journal the previous week shares with the group how they did and what they noticed about the journaling of other members. Often, members who have hit a "plateau" or have slipped from the program will volunteer to do the group journal as a way of getting "back on track."

14. Overeaters Anonymous meeting leaders are all volunteers, and there are no requirements other than willingness and at least a year of abstinence. Leaders

will usually serve a given meeting for an extended period of time and then seek out another volunteer as their replacement. The Serenity Prayer is this: "God grant me the serenity to accept the things I cannot change, courage to change the things I can, and the wisdom to know the difference." See http://oa.org for the full text of the invitation and full descriptions of Overeaters Anonymous meeting formats.

15. Service positions include meeting leader, secretary, and so on.

16. In Overeaters Anonymous, new members are asked to find someone who "has something you want" and to consider asking that person to be a sponsor.

17. See http://oa.org for a listing of the twelve steps and twelve traditions of Overeaters Anonymous.

18. There are several Overeaters Anonymous splinter groups that continue to base their abstinence on earlier Overeaters Anonymous food plans, for example, "food addicts anonymous" and "grey-sheeters anonymous."

19. This is similar to Mariana Valverde's characterization of the Alcoholics Anonymous approach to conceptualizing alcoholism as a "disease of the will" (Valverde 1998).

20. See "Our Invitation to You" on Overeaters Anonymous website, http://oa.org.

21. See Overeaters Anonymous website, http://oa.org, for an outline of the twelve steps.

22. Though most Overeaters Anonymous meetings are open to anyone, some cater to specific interest groups. There are meetings for gays and lesbians, women, African Americans, teens, and people who have lost or need to lose at least 100 pounds. While these meetings are generally open to all, they focus on the issues seen as most central to a given group.

23. All of the Overeaters Anonymous meetings I attended had a no cross-talk rule. This rule prohibits people from commenting on other people's "shares" or comments. The idea behind this rule, which is announced at the start of a meeting, is that people should be able to share without fear of the criticism or judgment they have so often experienced from doctors, diet groups, families, and others. Given this, in meetings, it is often hard to gauge the feelings of those who are listening to any speaker.

24. On the Overeaters Anonymous list serve, members are asked not to mention specific foods and, if they must, to include "food mentioned" in the subject line of their e-mail message. This is in consideration to those who are abstaining from any of the foods that may get mentioned. Newer members often have to be told this when they mention specific foods in their introductory e-mails.

25. The principle of anonymity is central to Overeaters Anonymous, as it is to other twelve-step programs. Therefore, all of the personal stories and testimonials published in official Overeaters Anonymous literature are credited to "anonymous." In meetings and online, members use their first names only. The principle of anonymity is meant to make people feel safe in honestly sharing their

experiences. A second meaning of the principle of anonymity is most clearly articulated in tradition twelve of the "12 Traditions of Overeaters Anonymous," in which anonymity is "the spiritual foundation of all these traditions, ever reminding us to place principles before personalities" (Overeaters Anonymous 1993, 249). In keeping with this sense, people do not share their personal stories in meetings or publications for personal recognition but to share Overeaters Anonymous principles and the program with others.

26. You can tell a fat compulsive overeater by looking at them, but you can't necessarily visually identify a thin or average compulsive overeater. This is of consequence when Overeaters Anonymous members do various forms of non–Overeaters Anonymous–sanctioned outreach. Though most members don't actively try to recruit people to Overeaters Anonymous, many share their experiences with friends, family, and coworkers whom they feel may suffer from the disease. In a more extreme case, one woman says that she carries pamphlets around with her and gives them to people she thinks are compulsive overeaters, and because she is talking with total strangers, most of the people she gives pamphlets to are fat. Though most Overeaters Anonymous members don't approach strangers to tell them about Overeaters Anonymous, many express a desire to do this when they see someone they feel might be a compulsive overeater.

CHAPTER 4   BYPASSING BLAME

1. The ASMBS is recognized by the American College of Surgeons and is a specialty surgical society in the Specialty and Service section of the American Medical Association. See notes in chapter 1 for more of the history of this organization.

2. Many people whose insurance will not cover the cost of weight-loss surgery go to another country, most often Mexico, to have the procedure done at a lower cost. While there are no data available on the number of such surgeries, several list serves, message boards, and even travel companies cater to such patients. For more on plastic surgery tourism see Gilman 2001.

3. According to the ASMBS, there are not yet any accurate statistics on the racial and ethnic backgrounds of weight-loss surgery patients. However, unlike plastic surgeries, most Roux-en-Y procedures are paid for by private insurance, Medicare, or Medicaid, thus potentially diversifying the class, racial, and ethnic composition of those who have or will have weight-loss surgery.

4. It is difficult to find outcome data on weight-loss surgeries as there are not yet any controlled clinical studies of the surgeries (see Buchwald et al. in *JAMA* October 2004). It is also the case that the studies that are available do not include long-term (five years or more) data on surgery outcomes.

5. As of 2010, Wilson has regained most of her surgically lost weight and has again embraced her body at a larger size.

6. For surgery to be approved by insurance companies as well as doctors, it is required that patients be able to document having tried and failed at traditional weight-loss methods.

7. It is generally accepted that the first nine to twelve months following gastric-bypass surgery is the "weight-loss window," the period when the vast majority of postoperative weight loss occurs.

8. "Dumping syndrome" is experienced by most RNY post-ops. The syndrome consists of weakness, nausea, sweats, vomiting, diarrhea, cramps, and fainting. Dumping is most often caused by eating high-sugar foods but can be caused by a wide variety of foods depending on the individual. The phenomenon is fully described in an informational pamphlet called *Understanding Obesity Surgery* (published by the Stay Well Company, a multimedia medical publications company) that is often given to post-op patients. People I spoke with often welcomed dumping as a type of aversion therapy, and some expressed missing it when, after two or more years post-op, they no longer experienced dumping.

9. The term *loser* is often used by weight-loss surgery patients to jokingly refer to themselves postsurgery. I also heard the term used at Weight Watchers, but it was far more common in the weight-loss surgery community.

10. In hospitals with specific bariatric surgery programs, patients are far more likely to be seen by a bariatric nurse than by their actual surgeon.

11. Most surgeons advise that weight-loss surgery patients have extensive blood work done every six months post-op in order to check for nutritional deficiencies common in RNY patients, including anemia and vitamin B_{12} deficiency.

12. Another reason for this is that after surgery the tendency to see surgical problems and failure to lose weight as a result of patient noncompliance again creates a doctor-patient relationship that patients would prefer to avoid.

13. Though there are certainly lesbians and gays who have had weight-loss surgery, all of my informants identified themselves as heterosexual.

14. Though the dividing line between "normal" and "plus-sizes" is arbitrary, the latter is generally considered to start at a 14/16 and extend to a 26/28. Most plus-size clothing stores carry items in this range; "women's" sections in major department stores generally end at a 24. For women needing larger sizes, their only option is to shop from websites or mail-order catalogs that specialize in "super-size" clothing.

15. The American Society of Plastic Surgeons estimates that in 2003 more than fifty-two thousand plastic surgeries were performed on postoperative bariatric surgery patients. The most popular procedures for bariatric patients are tummy tucks, panniculuctomies (removal of excess abdominal skin), breast reductions, calf lifts, breast lifts, lower body lifts, and upper arm lifts. (For more information go to http://www.plasticsurgery.org.)

16. Grabbing a beer with the guys while women shop might even more closely reproduce the heteronormative script evoked by Jeb, but people who have had weight-loss surgery are discouraged from drinking alcohol and carbonated beverages: the former because it is far more rapidly absorbed into the bloodstream postsurgery and the latter because the bubbles in carbonated beverages can contribute to "pouch stretching."

17. My interviewees point out that, for men, respect and recognition in society is not as appearance-based as it is for women. They all suggest that men don't have weight-loss surgery at the same rate as women because they do not suffer the same negative social consequences of obesity until they are at much higher relative weights.

18. For more on the framing of weight-loss as transformative, see Torrens 1998.

19. Compression garments are popular among post-op patients, especially those who have not yet had or cannot afford to have plastic surgery to remove "redundant skin." The garments range from compression panties to full body stockings that cover the body from the ankles to the wrists and neck. There are even compression masks to wear while sleeping. Many of these garments are produced and marketed specifically to the weight-loss surgery community. One woman I spoke to at the Obesity Help convention referred to her body stocking as "lipo in a box."

20. In my research I never encountered a speaker at a convention, support group, or information session who was more than five years post-op.

21. "2nd time around" refers to those patients who are going through weight-loss surgery revisions, a new surgery to rebuild the pouch and to attempt to narrow the stoma from the first surgery. Such procedures are often difficult to get approved by insurers as they carry added risks, and, indeed, many doctors will not perform such surgeries due to the increased risk of complications and death.

22. It is also the case that support groups, both in person and online, are a prime locus of the extension of the clinical gaze beyond the doctor and the clinic. In these groups, the "gaze" passes not only from doctor to patient, but from patient to patient, in some senses serving as a Foucauldian confessional in which the "truth" of weight-loss surgery is produced and disseminated (Foucault 1998, 1977; Spitzack 1990; Turner 1994).

23. This suggestion is particularly difficult to follow. Weight-loss surgery patients are required to drink a minimum of sixty-four ounces of water daily to prevent dehydration that can result from bypassing parts of the intestines. However, at the rate of one ounce every five minutes and not drinking with meals or for a time period before or after meals, patients would need to drink one ounce of fluid every five minutes for five and a half hours (not including mealtimes) every day just to take in the minimum amount of liquid recommended.

24. Because there are no scientific studies that evaluate the results of weight-loss surgery in those who are five years or more post-op, there is no way to accurately know rates of regain. The surgeon described above estimates (he did not cite any specific data) that after five years approximately 30 percent of RNY patients will have regained most, all, or more than their lost weight.

25. In a person who has RNY surgery and whose pouch was not made "too large" or whose pouch has not stretched, being able to eat a whole small hamburger would be unusual.

26. "Grazing" is a term used in the weight-loss surgery community for the eating of small bits of food all day long, rather than sticking to the three small meals they are supposed to eat. Often, when people are having trouble with postsurgery weight gain, the first question asked of them by their surgeon and their peers is, "Are you grazing?"

27. The diary was published on the Optifast website (www.optifast.com); however, since she has broken ties with the company, the journal has been removed.

CONCLUSION

1. The Association for Size Diversity and Health (ASDAH) has service marked the phrase "Health at Every Size" and is currently applying for a registered mark.

2. A full explanation of the HAES paradigm can be found at http://www.jonrobison .net/size.html (accessed January 5, 2012).

3. First published as the *Healthy Weight Journal* (until 2000), the *Health at Every Size Journal* was published by Gurze Books until fall 2006. Back issues can be found at http://www.bulimia.com/client/client_pages/haespdfs.cfm (accessed January 5, 2012).

4. Such research is not new; scientists have long been publishing research that questions accepted views of the relationship between weight and health, the value of ideal weights, and the efficacy of dieting (Bennett and Gurin 1992; Ernsberger and Haskew 1987; Knapp 1983). However, these early books and articles did not necessarily seek to advance a new paradigm of weight as does HAES. It is also the case that as little as ten to fifteen years ago obesity research did not have nearly the scientific clout and funding it does today in the midst of the epidemic; thus, those offering an alternative view of obesity were perhaps not as marginalized as those who question the existence and legitimacy of the obesity epidemic.

5. Indeed, there is an Internet group dedicated to the interpretation of mainstream obesity research and made up of HAES professionals from a number of different disciplines. Members help each other deconstruct many headline-making studies and provide each other with information about the methodological flaws frequently present in such studies, as well as how different methods of analyzing the same data might yield very different results. For example, a recent study published in the *Archive of Pediatric Adolescent Medicine* on the prevalence of diabetes (both type 1 and type 2 diabetes) in adolescents reported that adolescents with a BMI greater than the 85th percentile of all adolescents had a 2 percent chance of having impaired fasting glucose level (a sign of diabetes) than those adolescents with a BMI less than the 85th percentile, who had a 1 percent chance of impaired levels. The published study thus reports that fat adolescents have a 100 percent higher incidence of impaired fasting blood glucose levels than thinner adolescents. When this study was discussed on the list, it was pointed out that the findings also showed (but deemphasized) that, among adolescents of all sizes, 98 to 99 percent had normal fasting glucose

levels. Thus, while the 100 percent greater incidence figure reported in the study was technically true, the also-true observation that 98 to 99 percent of adolescents have normal blood glucose levels paints a far different and less catastrophic picture. Of course, as with the BMI, the blood glucose levels used to diagnose diabetes have also been revised downward in recent years (after the data used in this study was collected). This, combined with increased testing of youth and fat people, accounts for much of the frequently cited large increase in adult-onset diabetes in the past several years (Campos 2004).

6. The study was also funded in part by the California Cancer Research Grant and the California Agricultural Experiment Station.

7. Gynecological cancers include cancer of the breast, uterus, cervix, and ovary.

8. This effort on the part of HAES researchers to show the impact of size discrimination and fat phobia on the physical health of fat people while controlling for socioeconomic status, education, and race takes its cues from earlier studies that showed the impact of racism on the health status of African Americans.

APPENDIX

1. The limitations of and power embedded in language are also evident in my own use of terms to describe body weight. In general, I use quotation marks around the words *overweight* and *obesity* because these two terms are often decontextualized and naturalized as entities that are simply a matter of scientific fact. However, both terms have a social history, "obesity" as a disease category and medical term, and "overweight" as a normative term that implies that there is some objective weight that a person should not be "over." I make liberal use of the term "fat," which, while certainly not value-neutral, is a descriptive term and one that is often used by those who espouse a more critical, constructionist perspective on the obesity epidemic. I also use the term "above-average weight," which, while somewhat cumbersome, nonetheless does not as clearly assume a "normal" weight or presume a disease state.

2. These articles were culled from Lexis-Nexis and based on the presence of the term "obesity" in the headline or lead paragraph.

3. Most of my interviewees had been trying to lose weight for many years and have tried many different methods. Therefore, several interviewees have experience with both Overeaters Anonymous and Weight Watchers. I have categorized interviews based on which program an informant was currently active in.

4. The vast majority of Overeaters Anonymous meetings are open to the public; however, there are meetings geared toward certain groups of members, namely, survivors of sexual abuse, which are members-only meetings. I attended only meetings that were open to the public.

5. All of the support groups and informational seminars I attended were free and open to the public. The Obesity Help convention was also open to the public with payment of a sixty-dollar registration fee. As I discuss later, the Internet is

a main avenue of information, support, and community for those who have had or are interested in weight-loss surgery. *Obesity Help Magazine* is published six times a year by the organization ObesityHelp.com. Both the magazine and the website (http://www.ObesityHelp.com) are promoted as "your gateway to the weight-loss surgery community." ObesityHelp.com is a for-profit Internet community started in 1998. ObesityHelp.com offers online resources for weight-loss surgery patients, those considering surgery, surgeons, primary-care physicians, insurers, and more. The organization currently claims more than 250,000 members, most of them post-operative weight-loss surgery patients.

REFERENCES

Abbott, A. 1988. *The System of Professions: An Essay on the Division of Expert Labor.* Chicago: University of Chicago Press.

American Obesity Association (AOA). 1998. *Obesity: Increasing the Understanding of a Neglected Public Health Hazard.* Washington, DC: American Obesity Association.

———. 2000. *Objectives for Achieving and Maintaining a Healthy Population.* Washington, DC: American Obesity Association.

Amy, Nancy K., Annette E. Aalborg, Pat Lyons, and Laura Keranen. 2006. "Barriers to Routine Gynecological Cancer Screening for White and African-American Obese Women." *International Journal of Obesity* 30: 147–55.

Angier, Natalie. 2000. "Who Is Fat? It Depends on Culture." *New York Times*, November 7: F1–2.

Bacon, Linda. 2008. *Health at Every Size: The Surprising Truth About Your Weight.* Dallas: BenBella Books.

Barker, Kristin. 2005. *The Fibromyalgia Story: Medical Authority and Women's Worlds of Pain.* Philadelphia: Temple University Press.

Becker, Howard. 1963. *Outsiders: Studies in the Sociology of Deviance.* New York: Free Press.

Bennett, William, and Joel Gurin. 1992. *The Dieter's Dilemma.* New York: HarperCollins.

Boero, Natalie. 2007. "All the News That's Fat to Print: The American 'Obesity Epidemic' and the Media." *Qualitative Sociology* 3, no. 1: 41–61.

———. 2009. "Fat Kids, Working Moms, and the 'Epidemic of Obesity': Race, Class, and Mother-Blame." In *The Fat Studies Reader*, edited by Esther Rothblum and Sondra Solovay, 113–20. New York: New York University Press.

———. 2010. "Bypassing Blame: Bariatric Surgery and the Case of Biomedical Failure." In *Biomedicalization: Technoscience, Health, and Illness in the U.S.*, edited by Adele E. Clarke, Laura Mamo, Jennifer R. Fosket, Jennifer R. Fishman, and Janet K. Shim, 307–30. Durham, NC: Duke University Press.

Boero, Natalie, and C. J. Pascoe. Forthcoming. "Bringing the Pro-Ana Body Online: Pro-Anorexia Communities and Online Interaction." *Body and Society.*

Bordo, Susan. 1993. *Unbearable Weight: Feminism, Western Culture, and the Body.* Berkeley: University of California Press.

Braziel, Jana E. 2001. "Sex and Fat Chicks: Deterritorializing the Fat Female Body." In *Bodies out of Bounds: Fatness and Transgression*, edited by Jana Evans Braziel and Kathleen LeBesco, 231–56. Berkeley: University of California Press.

Brody, Jane. 1980. *Jane Brody's Nutrition Book*. New York: W. W. Norton and Company.

———. 1995. "Moderate Weight Gain Risky for Women, a Study Warns." *New York Times*, September 14: A1, B13.

———. 2000a. *The New York Times Book of Women's Health: The Latest on Feeling Fit, Eating Right, and Staying Well*. New York: Lebhar-Friedman Books.

———. 2000b. "Fat but Fit: A Myth about Obesity Is Slowly Being Debunked." *New York Times*, October 24: F7.

Buchwald, Henry, Yoav Avidor, Eugene Braunwald, Michael Jensen, Walter Pories, Kyle Farbach, and Karen Schoelles. 2004. "Bariatric Surgery: A Systematic Review and Meta-analysis. *Journal of the American Medical Association* 292, no. 14: 1724–37.

Burros, Marian. 1994a. "Despite Awareness of Risks, More in U.S. Are Getting Fat." *New York Times*, July 17: 1, 16.

———. 1994b. "Former Surgeon General Begins Push for Americans to Slim Down." *New York Times*, December 5: A20.

Campos, Paul. 2004. *The Obesity Myth: Why America's Obsession with Weight Is Hazardous for Your Health*. New York: Gotham Books.

Chang, Virginia W., and Nicholas A. Christakis. 2002. "Medical Modelling of Obesity: A Transition from Action to Experience in a 20th Century American Medical Textbook." *Sociology of Health & Illness* 24, no. 2 (March): 151–77.

Chapman, Gwen. 1999. "From 'Dieting' to 'Healthy Eating': An Exploration of Shifting Constructions of Eating for Weight Control." In *Interpreting Weight: The Social Management of Fatness and Thinness*, edited by Jeffery Sobal and Donna Maurer, 73–88. New York: Aldine de Gruyter.

Chernin, Kim. 1994. *The Hungry Self: Women, Eating, and Identity*. New York: Harper-Perinnial.

Chrisler, Joan C. 1996. "Politics and Women's Weight." *Feminism and Psychology* 6, no. 2: 181–84.

Clarke, Adele, Janet Shim, Laura Mamo, Jennifer Fosket, and Jennifer Fishman. 2003. "Biomedicalization: Technoscientific Transformations of Health, Illness, and US Biomedicine." *American Sociological Review* 68: 161–94.

Cohen, Stanley. 1972. *Folk Devils and Moral Panics*. New York: Routledge.

Conrad, Peter. 1992. "Medicalization and Social Control." *Annual Review of Sociology*, 209–32.

———. 2007. *The Medicalization of Society: On the Transformation of Human Conditions into Treatable Disorders*. Baltimore: Johns Hopkins University Press.

Conrad, Peter, and Joseph Schneider. 1992. *Deviance and Medicalization: From Badness to Sickness*. Philadelphia: Temple University Press.

Craddock, Susan. 1995. "Sewers and Scapegoats: Spatial Metaphors of Smallpox in the Nineteenth-Century San Francisco." *Social Science & Medicine* 41, no. 7: 957–68.

Crister, Greg. 2003. *Fat Land: How Americans Became the Fattest People in the World*. New York: Penguin.

Department of Health, Education, and Welfare (DHEW). 1979. *Healthy People: The Surgeon General's Report on Health Promotion and Disease Prevention*. Washington, DC: U.S. Public Health Service.

Department of Health and Human Services (DHHS). 1992. *Healthy People 2000: National Health Promotion and Disease Prevention Objectives.* 2nd ed. Boston: Jones and Bartlett Publishers.

———. 1998. *Leading Health Indicators for Healthy People 2010: Report from the HHS Working Group on Sentinel Objectives.* Washington, DC: U.S. Department of Health and Human Services, Office of Disease Prevention and Health Promotion.

———. 2002. *Healthy People 2010.* 2nd ed. McLean: International Medical Publishing.

———. 2010. *Healthy People 2010: Leading Health Indicators Priorities for Action.* http://www.healthypeople.gov/2010/LHI/Priorities.htm; accessed July 26, 2011.

DeVault, Majorie. 1991. *Feeding the Family: The Social Organization of Caring as Gendered Work.* Chicago: University of Chicago Press.

Dew, Kevin. 1999. "Epidemics, Panic, and Power: Representations of Measles and Measles Vaccines." *Health* 3, no. 4: 379–98.

Dull, Diana, and Candace West. 1991. "Accounting for Cosmetic Surgery: The Accomplishment of Gender." *Social Problems* 31: 801–17.

Eckerman, Lillian. 1994. "Foucault, Embodiment, and Gendered Subjectivities: The Case of Voluntary Self-Starvation." In *Foucault, Health, and Medicine,* edited by Alan Peterson and Robin Burton, 151–69. London: Routledge.

Ehrenreich, Barbara, and Deirdre English. 1978. *For Her Own Good: 150 Years of the Experts' Advice to Women.* New York: Doubleday.

Epstein, Steven. 1995. *Impure Science: Aids, Activism, and the Politics of Knowledge.* Berkeley: University of California Press.

Ernsberger, Paul, and Paul Haskew. 1987. *Rethinking Obesity: An Alternative View of Its Health.* New York: Human Sciences Press.

Farmer, Paul. 1999. *Infections and Inequalities: The Modern Plagues.* Berkeley: University of California Press.

Farrell, Amy. 2011. *Fat Shame: Stigma and the Fat Body in American Culture.* New York: New York University Press.

Fernandez, Don. 2008. "Alabama 'Obesity Penalty' Stirs Debate: Plan Calls for State Employees to Pay More for Health Insurance If They Don't Lose Weight." http://www.webmd.com/diet/news/20080825/alabama-obesity-penalty-stirs-debate; accessed August 25, 2008.

Ferris, Julie. 2003. "Parallel Discourses and 'Appropriate' Bodies: Media Constructions of Anorexia and Obesity in the Cases of Tracey Gold and Carnie Wilson." *Journal of Communication Inquiry* 27, no. 3 (July): 256–74.

Finkelstein, Eric A., and Laurie Zuckermann. 2008. *The Fattening of America: How the Economy Makes Us Fat, If It Matters, and What to Do about It.* Hoboken, NJ: John Wiley and Sons.

Foucault, Michel. 1977. *Discipline and Punish: The Birth of the Prison.* New York: Vintage Books.

———. 1994. *The Birth of the Clinic: An Archaeology of Medical Perception.* New York: Vintage.

———. 1997. *Society Must Be Defended: Lectures at the College De France, 1975–1976.* New York: Picador.

———. 1998. *The History of Sexuality,* Vol. 1: *An Introduction.* New York: Vintage Books.

Fraser, Laura. 1998. *Losing It: False Hopes and Fat Profits in the Diet Industry*. New York: Plume.

Freudenheim, Milt. 1999. "Employers Focus on Weight as Workplace Health Issue." *New York Times*, September 6: A15.

Fritsch, Jane. 1999. "Scientists Unmask Diet Myth: Willpower." *New York Times*, October 5: F1, F9.

Gaesser, Glenn. 2002. *Big Fat Lies: The Truth about Your Weight and Your Health*. Carlsbad, CA: Gurze Books.

Gamson, Joshua. 1991. "Silence, Death, and the Invisible Enemy: AIDS Activism and Social Movement 'Newness.'" In *Ethnography Unbound: Power and Resistance in the Modern Metropolis*, edited by Michael Burawoy, Alice Burton, Ann Arnett Fergusen, and Kathryn Fox, 35–57. Berkeley: University of California Press.

Gibbons, Michael Christopher, ed. 2008. *Ehealth Solutions for Healthcare Disparities*. New York: Springer.

Gilman, Sander. 2001. *Making the Body Beautiful: A Cultural History of Aesthetic Surgery*. Princeton, NJ: Princeton University Press.

Gitlin, Todd. 1980. *The Whole World Is Watching: Mass Media in the Making and Unmaking of the New Left*. Berkeley: University of California Press.

Glassner, Barry. 2000. *The Culture of Fear: Why Americans Are Afraid of the Wrong Things*. New York: Basic Books.

Goldberg, Carey. 2000. "Fat People Say an Intolerant World Condemns Them on First Sight." *New York Times*, November 5: A36.

Goode, Erica. 2000. "Watching Volunteers, Experts Seek Clues to Eating Disorders." *New York Times*, October 24: F1, F6.

Goode, Erich, and Nachman Ben-Yehuda. 1994. *Moral Panics: The Social Construction of Deviance*. Oxford: Blackwell.

Goodman, W. Charisse. 1995. *The Invisible Woman: Confronting Weight Prejudice in America*. Carlsbad, CA: Gurze Books, 1995.

Grady, Denise. 2000. "Exchanging Obesity's Risks for Surgery's." *New York Times*, October 12: A1, A26.

Grosz, Elizabeth A. 1994. *Volatile Bodies: Towards a Corporeal Feminism*. Bloomington: Indiana University Press.

Hatty, Suzanne E., and James Hatty. 1999. *The Disordered Body, Epidemic Disease, and Cultural Transformation*. Albany: SUNY Press.

Hill Collins, Patricia. 1990. *Black Feminist Thought: Knowledge, Consciousness, and the Politics of Empowerment*. New York: Routledge.

Hobson, Janell. 2003. "The 'Batty' Politic: Toward an Aesthetic of the Black Female Body." *Hypatia* 18, no. 4: 87–105.

hooks, bell. 2003. "Selling Hot Pussy: Representations of Black Female Sexuality in the Cultural Marketplace." In *The Politics of Women's Bodies: Sexuality, Appearance, and Behavior*, edited by Rose Weitz, 122–31. New York: Oxford University Press.

Hochschild, Arlie. 1989. *The Second Shift: Working Parents and the Revolution at Home*. New York: Viking Press.

Hubbard, V. S. 2000. "Defining Obesity and Overweight: What Are the Issues?" *American Journal of Clinical Nutrition* 72, no. 5: 1067–68.

Institutes of Medicine (IOM). 1998. *Leading Health Indicators for Healthy People 2010: First Interim Report*. Washington, DC: National Academy Press.

———. 1999a. *Leading Health Indicators for Healthy People 2010: Second Interim Report*. Washington, DC: National Academy Press.

———. 1999b. *Leading Health Indicators for Healthy People 2010: Final Report*. Washington, DC: National Academy Press.

Jutel, Annemarie. 2005. "Weighing Healthy: The Moral Burden of Obesity." *Social Semiotics* 15, no. 2: 113–25.

Kaiser Permanente. 2003. *Patient Information Booklet: Gastric Bypass Surgery*. Richmond, CA: Kaiser Permanente.

Kessler, David. 2009. *The End of Overeating: Taking Control of the Insatiable American Appetite*. New York: Rodale Books.

Kirkland, Anna. 2008. *Fat Rights: Dilemmas of Difference and Personhood*. New York: New York University Press.

———. 2011. "The Environmental Account of Obesity: A Case for Feminist Skepticism." *Signs: Journal of Women in Culture and Society* 36, no. 2 (Winter): 411–36.

Kirkland, Anna, and Jonathan Metzl. 2010. *Against Health: How Health Became the New Morality*. New York: New York University Press.

Klein, Richard. 1998. *Eat Fat*. New York: Vintage Books.

Knapp, Thomas R. 1983. "A Methodological Critique of the 'Ideal Weight' Concept." *Journal of the American Medical Association* 250, no. 4: 506–10.

Kolata, Gina. 2000a. "How the Body Knows When to Gain or Lose." *New York Times*, October 17: F1, F8.

———. 2000b. "Days Off Are Not Allowed, Weight Experts Argue." *New York Times*, October 18: A1, A26.

———. 2000c. "While Children Grow Fatter, Experts Search for Solutions." *New York Times*, October 19: A1, A26.

———. 2003. *Ultimate Fitness: The Quest for Truth about Health and Exercise*. New York: Farrar, Straus and Giroux.

———. 2008. *Rethinking Thin: The New Science of Weight Loss—and the Myths and Realities of Dieting*. New York: Farrar, Straus and Giroux.

Kolbert, Elizabeth. 2009. "XXXL: Why Are Americans So Fat?" *New Yorker*, http://www.newyorker.com/arts/critics/books/2009/07/20/090720crbo_books_kolbert; accessed July 20, 2009.

Kuczmarski, Robert, and Katherine Flegal. 2000. "Criteria for Definition of Overweight in Transition: Background and Recommendations for the United States." *American Journal of Clinical Nutrition* 72: 1074–81.

Lantz, Paula, and Karen Booth. 1998. "The Social Construction of the Breast Cancer Epidemic." *Social Science & Medicine* 46: 907–18.

Laqueur, Thomas W. 1992. *Making Sex: Body and Gender from Greeks to Freud*. Cambridge, MA: Harvard University Press.

Latour, Bruno. 1987. *Science in Action*. Cambridge, MA: Harvard University Press.

LeBesco, Kathleen. 2004. *Revolting Bodies? The Struggle to Redefine Fat Identity*. Amherst: University of Massachusetts Press.

———. 2010. "Fat Panic and the New Morality." In *Against Health: How Health Became the New Morality*, edited by Anna Kirkland and Jonathan Metzl, 72–83. New York: New York University Press.

Lester, Rebecca. 1999. "Let Go and Let God: Religion and the Politics of Surrender in Overeaters Anonymous." In *Interpreting Weight: The Social Management of Fatness and Thinness*, edited by Jeffrey Sobal and Donna Maurer, 139–64. New York: Aldine de Gruyter.

Lombardi, Kate Stone. 1997. "Treating Child Obesity: From Healthy Eating to Working Out." *New York Times*, July 20: WC1, WC7.

Lupton, Deborah. 1994. "Foucault and the Medicalisation Critique." In *Foucault, Health, and Medicine*, edited by Alan Peterson and Robin Bunton, 93–112. London: Routledge.

———. 1996. *Food, the Body, and the Self.* London: Sage.

Marcus, Frances Frank. 1998. "Why Baked Catfish Holds Lessons for Their Hearts." *New York Times*, June 21: WH24.

Marketdata Enterprises. 2009. *The U.S. Weight Loss & Diet Control Market.* Tampa, FL: Lynbrook.

Martin, Emily. 1987. *The Woman in the Body: A Cultural Analysis of Reproduction.* Boston: Beacon Press.

Mehra, Beloo. 2008. "Research or Personal Quest: Dilemmas in Studying My Own Kind." In *Multiple and Intersecting Identities in Qualitative Research*, edited by Betty Marie Merchant and Arlette Ingram Willis, 79–94. Oxford: Taylor & Francis e-Library.

Merton, Robert K. 1972. "Insiders and Outsiders: A Chapter in the Sociology of Knowledge." *American Journal of Sociology* 78 (July): 9–47.

Metzl, Jonathan. 2010. "Introduction, Why 'Against Health'?" In *Against Health: How Health Became the New Morality*, edited by Anna Kirkland and Jonathan Metzl, 1–15. New York: New York University Press.

Millman, Marcia. 1980. *Such a Pretty Face: Being Fat in America.* New York: Berkeley Books.

Mink, Gwendolyn. 1995. *The Wages of Motherhood: Inequality in the Welfare State, 1917–1942.* Ithaca, NY: Cornell University Press.

Moon, Dawne. 2004. *God, Sex, and Politics: Homosexuality and Everyday Theologies.* Chicago: University of Chicago Press.

Mundy, Alicia. 2001. *Dispensing with the Truth: The Victims, the Drug Companies, and the Dramatic Story behind the Battle over Fen-Phen.* New York: St. Martin's Press.

National Heart, Lung, and Blood Institute (NHLBI). 2000. *The Practical Guide: Identification, Evaluation, and Treatment of Overweight and Obesity in Adults.* Washington, DC: National Institutes of Health.

———. 2011. *Calculate Your BMI.* http://nhlbisupport.com/bmi/; accessed July 26, 2011.

Negrin, Llewellyn. 2002. "Cosmetic Surgery and the Eclipse of Identity." *Body & Society* 8, no. 4: 21–42.

New York Times. 1994. "Trimming the Nation's Fat." December 11: E4.

———. 1997. "Virus May Lie behind Some Obesity." April 8: C6.

———. 1998. "U.S. to Widen Its Definition of Who Is Fat." June 4: A22.

Nidetch, Jean. 1972. *The Memoir of a Successful Loser: The Story of Weight Watchers*. New York: New American Library.

Obesity Help. 2004. "'These Are Better Days' for Carnie Wilson: Living Life with Lymphodema and Obesity." *Obesity Help* 5: 40–43.

Oliver, J. Eric. 2006. *Fat Politics: The Real Story behind America's Obesity Epidemic*. New York: Oxford University Press.

Orbach, Susie. 1978. *Fat IS a Feminist Issue*. New York: Berkeley Books.

Ortner, Sherry. 1986. "Is Female to Nature as Male Is to Culture?" In *Woman, Culture, and Society*, edited by Michelle Rosaldo and Louise Lamphere, 67–87. Palo Alto, CA: Stanford University Press.

Overeaters Anonymous. 1993. *The Twelve Steps and Twelve Traditions of Overeaters Anonymous*. California: Overeaters Anonymous.

Pascoe, C. J., and Natalie Boero. Under Contract. *Mias and Wannas: Community and Identity in a Pro-Ana Subculture*. Ann Arbor: University of Michigan Press.

Pollan, Michael. 2007. *The Omnivore's Dilemma: A Natural History of Four Meals*. New York: Penguin.

———. 2008. *In Defense of Food: An Eater's Manifesto*. New York: Penguin.

Poulton, Terry. 1997. *No Fat Chicks: How Big Business Profits by Making Women Hate Their Bodies—and How to Fight Back*. New York: Birch Lane Press.

Power, Michael L., and Jay Schulkin. 2009. *The Evolution of Obesity*. Baltimore: Johns Hopkins University Press.

Reissman, Catherine Kohler. 1983. "Women and Medicalization: A New Perspective." *Social Policy* 14: 3–18.

Rose, Nicholas. 1994. "Medicine, History, and the Present." In *Reassessing Foucault: Power, Medicine, and the Body*, edited by Colin Jones and Roy Porter, 48–72. London: Routledge.

Rosenberg, Charles. 1962. *The Cholera Years: The United States in 1832, 1849, and 1866*. Chicago: University of Chicago Press.

———. 1992. *Explaining Epidemics and Other Studies in the History of Medicine*. Cambridge: Cambridge University Press.

Rothblum, Esther. 1999. "Contradictions and Confounds in Coverage of Obesity: Psychology Journals, Textbooks, and Media." *Journal of Social Issues* 55: 355–69.

Rothblum, Esther, and Sondra Solovay. 2009. *The Fat Studies Reader*. New York: New York University Press.

Saguy, Abigail C., and Rene Almeling. 2008. "Fat in the Fire? Science, the News Media and the 'Obesity Epidemic.'" *Sociological Forum* 23, no. 1 (March): 55–83.

Saguy, Abigail C., and Paul Campos. 2011. "Medical and Scientific Debates over Obesity." In *Handbook of the Social Science of Obesity*, edited by John Cawley. New York: Oxford University Press.

Saguy, Abigail C., and Kjerstin Gruys. 2010. "Morality and Health: News Media Constructions of Overweight and Eating Disorders." *Social Problems* 57, no. 2 (November): 231–50.

Saguy, Abagail C., Kjerstin Gruys, and Shanna Gong. 2010. "Social Problem Construction and National Context: News Reporting on 'Overweight' and 'Obesity' in the United States and France." *Social Problems* 57, no. 4 (November): 586–610.

Saguy, Abigail C., and Anna Ward. 2011. "Coming Out as Fat: Rethinking Stigma." *Social Psychology Quarterly* (March): 53–75.

Salant, Tayla, and Heena Santry. 2006. "Internet Marketing of Bariatric Surgery: Contemporary Trends in the Medicalization of Obesity." *Social Science & Medicine* 62, no. 10: 2445–57.

Schlosser, Eric. 2005. *Fast Food Nation: The Darker Side of the All-American Meal.* New York: Harper Perennial.

Schrock, Douglas, Lori Reid, and Emily Boyd. 2005. "Transsexuals' Embodiment of Womanhood." *Gender and Society* 19, no. 3: 317–35.

Schwartz, Hillel. 1986. *Never Satisfied: A Cultural History of Diets, Fantasies, and Fat.* London: Collier Macmillan Publishers.

Shoenfielder, Lisa, and Barb Weiser. 1983. *Shadow on a Tightrope: Writings by Women on Fat Oppression.* San Francisco: Aunt Lute Books.

Showalter, Elaine. 1997. *Hystories: Hysterical Epidemics and Modern Media.* New York: Columbia University Press.

Shuter, Rob. 2010. "Carnie Wilson Doesn't Care If You Think She's Fat." *PopEater,* http://www.popeater.com/2010/12/10/wilson-phillips-carnie-weight-naughty-but-nice-with-rob/; accessed December 10, 2010.

Sobal, Jeffrey. 1995. "The Medicalization and Demedicalization of Obesity." In *Eating Agendas: Food and Nutrition as Social Problems,* edited by Donna Maurer and Jeffrey Sobal, 67–90. New York: Aldine de Gruyter.

———. 1999. "The Size Acceptance Movement and the Social Construction of Body Weight." In *Weighty Issues: Fatness and Thinness as Social Problems,* edited by Jeffrey Sobal and Donna Maurer, 231–49. New York: Aldine de Gruyter.

Solovay, Sondra. 2000. *Tipping the Scales of Justice: Fighting Weight-Based Discrimination.* Amherst, NY: Prometheus Books.

Spector, Malcolm, and John I. Kitsuse. 1977. *Constructing Social Problems.* Menlo Park: Cummings Press

Spitzack, Carol. 1990. *Confessing Excess: Women and the Politics of Body Reduction.* Albany: SUNY Press.

Starr, Paul. 1984. *The Social Transformation of American Medicine: The Rise of a Sovereign Profession and the Making of a Vast Industry.* New York: Basic Books.

Stearns, Peter. 1997. *Fat History: Bodies and Beauty in the Modern West.* New York: New York University Press.

Stimson, Karen. 1983. "Fat, Fitness, and Exercise—Health or Healthism?" *Ample Apple newsletter,* October, http://www.eskimo.com/~largesse/Archives/healthism.html; accessed August 3, 2011.

Stinson, Kandi. 2001. *Women and Dieting Culture: Inside a Commercial Weight Loss Group.* New Brunswick, NJ: Rutgers University Press.

Thomas, Pattie, and Carl Wilkerson. 2005. *Taking Up Space: How Eating Well and Exercising Regularly Saved My Life.* Nashville: Pearlsong Press.

Torrens, Kathleen. 1998. "I Can Get Any Job and Feel Like a Butterfly! Symbolic Violence in the TV Advertising of Jenny Craig." *Journal of Communication Inquiry* 22, no. 1: 27–47.

Treichler, Paula. 1999. *How to Have Theory in an Epidemic: Cultural Chronicles of AIDS.* Durham, NC: Duke University Press.

Turner, Bryan. 1994. "From Governmentality to Risk: Some Reflections on Foucault's Contribution to Medical Sociology." In *Foucault, Health, and Medicine,* edited by Alan Peterson and Robin Bunton, ix–xxi. London: Routledge.

University of Texas Health Science Center. 2005. "'U.S. Surgeon General Carmona Calls Obesity 'The Terror Within.'" http://www.uthscsa.edu/hscnews/singleformat2 .asp?newID=1381; accessed March 1, 2005.

Valverde, Mariana. 1998. *Diseases of the Will: Alcohol and the Dilemmas of Freedom.* New York: Cambridge University Press.

Wade, Nicholas. 1994. "Truly Gross Economic Product." *New York Times,* October 16: SM24.

Wann, Marilyn. 1998. *Fat! So? Because You Don't Have to Apologize for Your Size.* New York: Ten Speed Press.

Wansink, Brian. 2007. *Mindless Eating: Why We Eat More Than We Think.* New York: Bantam Dell.

West, Candace, and Don Zimmerman. 1987. "Doing Gender." *Gender and Society* 1: 125–51.

Williams, Lena. 1990. "Growing Up Flabby in America: Vain Attempts to Get Children in Shape." *New York Times,* March 22: C1, C6.

Winter, Greg. 2000. "Fraudulent Marketers Capitalize on Demand for Sweat-Free Diets." *New York Times,* October 29: A1, A26.

Wolf, Anne M., and Graham A. Colditz. 1998. "Current Estimates of the Economic Cost of Obesity in the United States." *Obesity Research* 6, no. 2: 97–106.

Zimberg, Robyn. 1993. "Food, Needs, and Entitlement: Women's Experience of Emotional Eating." In *Consuming Passions: Feminist Approaches to Weight Preoccupation and Eating Disorders,* edited by Catrina Brown and Karin, 137–51. Jasper, Toronto: Second Story Press.

Zola, Irving. 1972. "Medicine as an Institution of Social Control." *Sociological Review* 20: 487–504.

INDEX

ABOUT THE AUTHOR

NATALIE BOERO is an assistant professor of sociology at San Jose State University in San Jose, California. She received her PhD in sociology from the University of California at Berkeley in 2006 and has published in numerous journals and edited volumes on the topics of obesity, gender, health, and eating disorders.